NAET: SAY GOOD-BYE
TO YOUR ALLERGIES

DEVI S. NAMBUDRIPAD,

M.D., D.C., L.Ac., Ph.D. (Acu.)

Author of
Say Good-Bye to ... series

THIS BOOK WILL REVOLUTIONIZE
THE PRACTICE OF MEDICINE

The doctor of the future will give no medicine,
But will interest his patients
In the care of the human frame, in diet,
And in the cause and prevention of disease
-Thomas A. Edison

Published by
DELTA PUBLISHING COMPANY
6714 Beach Blvd.
Buena Park, CA 90621
(888) 890-0670, (714) 523-8900 Fax: (714) 523-3068
Web site: www.naet.com

DEDICATION

This book is dedicated to
patients suffering from
allergies of all types.

First Edition, 2003

Library of Congress Control No: 2002116895

ISBN: 0-9704344-3-X

Printed in U.S.A.

Table of Contents

ACKNOWLEDGEMENT

I am deeply grateful to my husband, Dr. Kris Nambudripad, for his encouragement and assistance in my schooling and, later, in the formulation of this project. Without his cooperation in researching reference work, revision of manuscripts, word processing and proofreading, it is doubtful whether this book would have ever been completed.

My sincere thanks also go to the many clients who have entrusted their care to me, for without them I would have had no case studies, no feedback, and certainly no extensive source of personal research upon which to base this book.

I am also deeply grateful to Mary Karaba, Karen Watts, Meg Brazil, Shirley Reason, Ileen Garcia, Joyce Baisden, Helene Singer, Lettie Vipond, Toby Weiss, Amy Clute, Michael Magrutsch, Karen Tuckerman, Rosemary Depauw, Margaret Davies, Dikran Ayarian, to name a few among many of my devoted patients, for believing in me from the very beginning of the research until the present, and by supporting my theory and helping me to conduct the ongoing detective work.

I also have to express my thanks to my son, Roy, who assisted me in many ways in the writing of this book. Roy was a one year old and very sick when I practiced my technique on him at the beginning of my search for an allergy cure. Now, he is a 22-year-old, healthy, levelheaded, responsible young man who is an outstanding medical student.

Additionally, I wish to thank Robert Prince, M.D., Dr. Vijay Pratap, Ph. D., Doretta Zemp, M.A., M.F., M.F.T., Barbara Levitt, Candace Smith, Chi Yu, Fong Tien and many of my associates who wish to remain anonymous for proofreading and assisting me with this work, and Mr. Sri at Delta Publishing for his printing expertise. I am deeply grateful for my professional training and the knowledge and skills acquired in classes and seminars on chiropractic and kinesiology at the Los Angeles College of Chiropractic in Whittier, California; the California Acupuncture College in Los Angeles; SAMRA University of Oriental Medicine, Los Angeles; University of Health Sciences, School of Medicine, Antigua; and the clinical experience received at the clinics attached to these colleges.

My special thanks also go to Mala Moosad, N.D., R.N., L.Ac., Mohan Moosad, M.S., N.D., D. Ac, who supported and stood by me from the very beginning of my NAET discovery and ongoing research. They helped immensely by taking over my work at the clinic so that I could complete the book. I also would like to acknowledge my thanks to my dear mother for nourishing me emotionally and nutritionally. My heartfelt thanks also go to Margaret Wu and Barbara Cesmat, NAET practitioners, who have dedicated their time to help desperate allergy sufferers by assisting me in many ways to promote my mission of making NAET available to every needy person in the universe. I would also like to acknowledge my everlasting thanks to my office manager, Janna Gossen, who worked with me from the first day of my practice almost two decades ago and to all the other staff members and all other NAET practitioners who support me and stand with me to help more allergic victims find health through NAET.

I would like to remember the late Dr. Richard F. Farquhar at Farquhar Chiropractic Clinic in Bellflower, California. I was a student of chiropractic and acupuncture when I was doing preceptorship with him. When I told him about my NAET discovery, he tried the treatment on himself and was amazed with the results. Then he encouraged me to practice NAET with needles on all his patients. Because of his generosity, I had the opportunity to treat hundreds of patients soon after I discovered NAET.

I am so delighted to express my sincere thanks to the Los Angeles College of Chiropractic for teaching different branches of holistic medicine like kinesiology and Sacro-occipital techniques along with chiropractic in our school and providing the students with a sound knowledge in nutrition. Because of that I was able to combine the art of kinesiology, chiropractic and nutrition along with acupuncture/acupressure and develop NAET. California Acupuncture College also taught me a few lessons in kinesiology along with the art and science of acupuncture. I do not have enough words to express my heartfelt thanks and appreciation to California Acupuncture State Board for supporting NAET from the beginning, permitting me to teach other licensed acupuncturists, by instantly making me a CEU provider soon after I discovered it. Perhaps the California Acupuncture State Board will never know how much they have helped humanity by validating my new technique and allowing me to share the treatment method with other practitioners and, through them, to the countless number of patients like me who now live a normal life. I am forever indebted to acupuncture and Oriental medicine. Without this knowledge, I, myself, would still be living in pain. Thank you for allowing me to share my experience with the world!

I also extend my sincere appreciation and thanks to my medical school professors for willing to part with their knowledge and help us become great physicians. I would like to extend my sincere thanks to these great teachers especially to my medical school mentors and professors from Antigua and from California, and the staff of the respective hospitals I did my clinicals. Without their guidance and teaching I doubt if I could have completed the medical school.

All my mentors from all professional schools I attended have helped me to grow immensely at all levels. They are also indirectly responsible for the improvement of my personal health as well as that of my family, patients, and the health of other NAET practitioners and their countless patients.

Many of my professors, doctors of Western and Oriental medicine, allopathy, chiropractic, kinesiology, as well as nutritionists, were willing to give of themselves by teaching and committing personal time, through interviews, to help me complete this book. I will always be eternally grateful to them. They demonstrated the highest ideals of the medical profession.

Devi S. Nambudripad, M.D., D.C., L.Ac., Ph.D.(Acu.)

FOREWORD
By
Robert Cohen, M.D.

As a medical doctor, I came into the NAET office first as a curious observer, then as a patient with seasonal allergies. My interest grew and soon I found myself not only taking introductory classes but also advanced NAET treatment classes because of the exceptional results I witnessed among my patients.

My background in medical research soon had me volunteering to assist in preliminary research studies as well as evaluating the multitude of case studies submitted by NAET practitioners worldwide. The one common denominator I found in the wide spectrum of patients treated was that no matter what the disorder is, whether a simple milk allergy patient or a more complex autistic child, NAET seemed to work. Practitioners got amazing results in heretofore-untreatable conditions.

The practice and theories of medicine today are different in many ways than those of 20 or even 10 years ago. Doctors, not satisfied with just dispensing pills, are evaluating the plethora of complementary approaches from many medical disciplines, both Eastern and Western. As physicians, we want answers and effective solutions to treat our difficult cases. Dr. Nambudripad, after years of research has incorporated her expertise from various medical fields to create this natural, truly integrative treatment technique called NAET. NAET combines theories from many medical fields to accurately interview, diagnose and treat patients. It is difficult to assign NAET into a specific medical field. If one were to classify it, the field would most appropriately be labeled "Energeticpsychoneuroimmunology."

Dr. Nambudripad is one of those rare physicians who dare to question commonly accepted treatment principles and improve upon them. She had the vision to clearly see the links between many divergent fields and "connect the dots." She once related to me, "It was always there in the books I read. I didn't do anything new. I just put it together." She has the tenacity and energy to continually improve her technique while treating patients and teaching other medical providers.

Now, as the Medical Research Director of Nambudripad's Allergy Research Foundation (NARF), I have been able to observe NAET from both the clinical side as well as from a more controlled scientific point of view. I have seen a patient with a seven- year history of clinically diagnosed asthma, who was taking three daily medications, complete NAET treatments and be symptom free. Mothers of severely autistic children have seen their children begin to focus, communicate and already improve after NAET treatments. Our controlled studies have demonstrated statistically significant improvements with a variety of substances. Our studies tested the efficacy of NAET on many food products including milk, garlic and eggs. Case studies by our worldwide network of practitioners have included dramatic improvements in arthritis, MS, diabetes, ADD, ADHD, OCD, migraine headaches, heart palpitations and hypertension, just to name a few. We have been encouraged by representatives from medical schools and the National Institute of Health to continue our research as they, too, are interested in NAET results. NAET truly stands on the forefront of a new evolution in the paradigm of medical diagnosis and treatment.

This book is for both the experienced NAET practitioner as well as the uninitiated. Both doctor and patient will gain a greater understanding of the concepts and philosophy behind the treatment technique that is NAET. Most importantly, it is for anyone who has a thirst for knowledge and a passion to help those in pain. Dr.

Nambudripad has tirelessly created the key to good health that will open the locks of illness for millions of sufferers and return them to a life of happiness and vitality.

Robert Cohen, M.D.
Director of NARF
Buena Park, California
January 2003

PREFACE

Since childhood I suffered from a multitude of health problems. Because of this prolonged and firsthand experience with ill health, I became focused on health-related problems, particularly those related to allergies; this, in turn, resulted in my natural inclination to pursue medicine as a profession. Consequently, I became a registered nurse, chiropractor, kinesiologist, acupuncturist and, later, a doctor of allopathic medicine, now an M.D. I began specializing in the treatment of the allergic patient, using methods I learned through an intensive study of Oriental medicine combined with the more traditional Western methods learned in various schools of Western medicine.

During my studies and early practice as an allergist, while using eclectic methods of allergy treatments, I discovered a technique that eliminated most of my health problems.

Integrating the relevant techniques from the various fields I studied, combined with my own discoveries, has become the focus of my practice.

There is no known successful method of treatment for food allergies using Western medicine except avoidance, which means deprivation and frustration. Each of the disciplines I studied provided bits of knowledge that I used in developing a new treatment to permanently eliminate allergies, which is now known throughout the world as Nambudripad's Allergy Elimination Techniques, or NAET for short.

As an infant, living in India, my birthplace, I had severe infantile eczema, which lasted until I was seven or eight years old. My eczema started at 11 months old after eating a whole tomato one night instead of dinner, as my mother recalled. After that, I was administered Western medicine, Ayurvedic herbal medicine, various cleansing diets without a break until I was eight years old. I was born and brought up as a vegetarian. From childhood, my major diet was organically grown vegetables - fruits and grains grown in our fields (without using any artificial or chemical fertilizers). My family was into farming. When I turned one year old, after the 'Tomato' dinner my health problems began one after another: First started as generalized skin rashes, hives, eczema, dermatitis, sinusitis, sinus troubles, angioneurotic edema (swelling in different body parts - frequently eyelids, face, sometimes even throat without any warning or known cause), and severe arthritis. My saga continued... frequent colds and fevers, flu-like symptoms, constant post nasal drip, thick mucus in the throat, pain and swelling in the joints, severe fatigue, and general body ache. By the time I was ten, I began having severe migraines, then later, severe PMS. I never had anything mild. My symptoms were always in extremes making living difficult. I spend my childhood visiting doctors and taking medicines, yet I still suffered constantly.

Ayurveda is the traditional Indian system of medicine based largely on herbs and naturopathy. This helped a bit. Ayurveda has certain rules to observe while one is taking those herbal concoctions. One's food is very limited to bland overcooked vegetables, and steamed rice for 14 days; then continue another 14 days with the same diet without any herbal drinks. Then another with light food (no fried food, spicy food, etc.) Every four months, 14-day herbal drink was repeated. Now when I look back, I can clearly see why I was doing well while I was on this herbal program — because I was just eating clean, bland, overcooked food. While I was taking the herbal medicines, my symptoms were controlled, but whenever I went off the herbs more than the four-month cycle, my eczema recurred. When I was eight years old, one of the herbal doctors told my parents to feed me only white rice cooked with a special herb formula. The major ingredients in this special blend included Coriander leaves, and dry Coriander seeds, among a few other minor herbs. (See the end notes for instruction on preparation of this rice-meal). Coriander is currently on the mind of all herbal doctors since the Japanese discovered that Coriander is a natural detoxifier for chemicals, pesticides, and mercury. According to Chinese medicine, Coriander leaves and the seeds have the property of liver fire cleansing and spleen chi tonification. That means they help improve the digestion and elimination of toxin.

This special diet helped me a great deal. The herbalist seemed to know what he was doing. In the village where I grew up, the village health department service engaged in spraying DDT weekly around the house and neighborhood to destroy mosquitoes and eradicate Malaria, the prevalent killer at that time in my village. It worked well to totally eradicate Malaria from the village, but some of the young, weak infants and children continued to suffer the consequences of pesticide poisoning for many years afterward.

After discovering NAET, treating myself and eliminating known allergens, pesticides still remained a big problem for me. I continued to treat each pesticide as they crossed my path. After treatment, the particular type did not bother me anymore. But I often wondered why I was so allergic to pesticides.

The mystery was solved when I visited my birthplace in 1995. My cousins and I decided to take a walk along the valley where we played as children, revisiting and refreshing the nostalgic memories of our old times. After we walked for about five minutes, one of my cousins looked at my face and let out a scream. My face had turned red, with huge hives all over my face and neck. My body was hot. I felt my legs go very weak, as if they would give up any minute. My lungs were working hard to get air. My cousins were scared, not knowing what was happening to me. I, too, was surprised at this sudden, unexpected reaction when I thought I had conquered all my allergies. We turned back. I leaned onto my cousin's shoulder to prevent falling.

Suddenly, I noticed some white patches on all the leaves and grasses on the ground, as if someone had sprayed diluted white paint all over.

"What is this?" I asked, pointing toward the white patches.

One of my cousins answered, "It is DDT. We have had some problems with mosquitoes lately, due to the new rubber plantations. The health department has been spraying DDT for months now every week. They had just sprayed this morning."

I sighed in relief. So again, pesticide-DDT was a culprit. I asked my cousin to collect some of the leaves. Once I reached the house, I quickly treated myself for DDT along with the leaves. In less than 10 minutes, my breathing became normal. In 40 minutes, all the hives disappeared. My body strength and leg strength returned. I became normal again. Thank you God, for granting me NAET.

I then remembered my young days in the valley. The cause of my illness could have been the DDT spray. I always felt fatigued and listless while I was there. It was a chore for me to get through the days, a chore to breathe. I suffered from dermatitis and eczema all my life until I treated myself with NAET. I suffered from chronic nasal allergies; sometimes from a runny nose, sometimes from completely blocked nostrils. I struggled with shortness of breath and coughs ever since I can remember.

After NAET, I do not suffer shortness of breath anymore, but I still suffer coughing spells with any irritation to my lungs. One of my recent lung scans revealed that I own congenital-emphysematous lungs. My pulmonologist couldn't believe that in spite of having such lungs, I still do very well; my respiratory tract works normally.

Personal and Professional Chronology

I got married and moved to Los Angeles in 1976. My husband had been suffering from some health problems and was following a strict diet under the supervision of a nutritionist. I became even more health-conscious, and tried to change my own eating habits by adding more fruits, vegetables, whole grain products and complex carbohydrates into my daily diet, under the advice of the same nutritionist. All of a sudden, I became very ill. One by one, I came down with bronchitis, pneumonia, and my arthritis returned. Then symptoms multiplied. I suffered from insomnia, clinical depression, constant sinusitis and frequent migraine headaches. I felt extremely tired all the time, but remained fully awake when I went to bed.

I tried many different antibiotics and medicines, changed doctors, and consulted more nutritionists. All the medication, vitamins, and herbs that I took made me sicker, and the consumption of good, whole foods made me worse.

Between 1976 and 1980, I had three miscarriages, which affected me emotionally. In order to keep my sanity, I decided to go back to school, coughing and puffing my way through. One might think I was a lifelong smoker or a T.B. patient! Following my mother's advice, I turned to God and began to observe all of my family's traditional religious holidays. I fasted, with only water intake on all the Hindu holy days. The day after a fast I would feel better, would have more energy, and my mind would be clearer. I became very religious. I know now that staying away from foods I was allergic to was the reason for my feeling of well being the next day of the fast. Of course, I know that God played a great role, too. According to the Hindu Bible "Gita," God, will only help you if you take the initiative to help yourself first. If you try and reach halfway, He will meet you there and travel with you the rest of the way. So by fasting, avoiding the allergenic foods, tirelessly attending schools after schools, discovering the allergy elimination techniques, eliminating my allergies and related illnesses, I had reached the halfway point on the journey to my destination.

In 1981, I started the acupuncture college. The very first class was on acupressure, entitled Touch for Health. The first day, my instructor taught muscle response testing, to detect food allergies. By then, my cough had returned. The teacher noticed my chronic, raspy cough, suspected I was suffering from food allergies, and tested me for various allergies to food items through muscle response testing. I reacted to almost everything except white rice and broccoli. He suggested that I might do better if I ate white rice and broccoli exclusively for a few days.

By that time I had been examined and treated by many doctors, including neurologists, cardiologists, psychologists, nutritionists and herbalists, but none suspected food allergies as a cause of my chronic ill health. I was excited by this new possibility. I was willing to try anything to get better. I followed my teacher's advice and ate white rice and broccoli exclusively. Within one week's time, my bronchitis cleared up, my nasal allergies were better, my headaches became infrequent and less intense, my joint pains eased, and my back ceased hurting. My thinking and concentration became clearer. My depression of two years disappeared, so did the insomnia. My general body aches cleared. For the first time in my life, I experienced pain-free days. Until then, I was under the impression that everybody was supposed to experience a certain amount of body aches and pains all the time because I had never known otherwise. It was a delight for me to go to bed without pain and wake up in the morning without pain.

After that week's restricted diet, I tried eating some other foods but my symptoms returned. I began eating only white rice and broccoli again.

I mentioned earlier that I was a strict vegetarian. After being on rice and overcooked broccoli, I noticed that I could not eat salads, fruits or vegetables, because, as I eventually discovered, I was very allergic to vitamin C. As we know, vitamin C is the most important vitamin in the body to keep the body in normal health. It is an antioxidant. It is important for taking care of wear and tear in the body. It is important to rejuvenate the cells by expelling toxins from the tissue and generating new cells. It is important for growth and development. Vitamin C is the basic component of collagen materials in the body. Collagen fibers are the building block for the muscles, ligaments and connective tissue. Vitamin C protects against infections and inflammations. My brain-computer software had a virus. According to my mother, when I was born I was perfect, and continued to be perfect until 11 months old. So something around that time caused the entry of the virus into my brain-computer and caused disruption of the software. I had vitamin C deficiency symptoms. Since I was a vegetarian, I was consuming plenty of vitamin C, but I did not absorb it. Since I was so allergic to vitamin C, cells could not function normally and eliminate the toxins produced in my body - my body became more and more toxic by the hour and the toxins began invading my entire body causing all systemic problems I mentioned before.

I could not eat all other foods that normal people eat because I was very allergic to all the nutrients. I could not eat whole grain products because they contained B complex; fruits, honey or any products made from sugars because I was very allergic to sugar; milk or milk products because I was very allergic to calcium; dark greens because I was allergic to vitamin A; egg products because I was allergic to all proteins and caused skin and joint problems. I was allergic to all types of dried beans, including soybeans, which gave me severe joint pains, sensation of heaviness in the head and backaches. Most spices, especially, the pepper family, gave me arthritis and migraines. Almost all fabrics, except silk, gave me itching problems, joint pain, and caused extreme tiredness. Before I met my teacher at the Acupuncture school, I thought I was going crazy and I was having psychosomatic problems. My teacher at the acupuncture college confirmed my doubts: I was simply allergic to almost everything under the sun, including the sun by heat and radiation.

It seemed that I was allergic to everything except white rice, broccoli, silk and aspirin. What a combination! At least I was lucky to have a few non-allergenic items. In my practice, I now see many less fortunate patients, people who have allergies to everything one could imagine. Most of them could live only in a bubble-like environment before they were treated with NAET.

One day in 1983, around 2 pm, I came home from school and found I didn't have any more cooked rice. I put on some rice to cook. While I was waiting for the rice to cook, I ate a few pieces of carrot. In just a few minutes, I felt tired and lethargic, like I was going to pass out. I immediately gave me an acupuncture treatment by inserting needles in many acupuncture points to prevent me from fainting. I fell asleep while in the acupuncture session. The rest is history. When I awoke I felt strangely different. I was not sick or tired anymore. Instead, I felt a renewed, pleasant energy.

Suddenly, I wondered whether there could be any connection between the acupuncture treatment while carrot touching my skin and my sudden sense of well-being. During that semester I was attending a class in electromagnetic field theory and acupuncture at the Oriental Medical College. This helped me understand the connection between the electromagnetic force of my body and the carrot. In class, we were taught that every object on earth, whether living or nonliving, possesses a surrounding electromagnetic energy field. Earth has its own energy field. Every object is attracted to Earth. Every object on earth is also attracted to one another. All these different energies can attract or repel from one another, depending upon their energy differences.

I then tested the carrot using muscle response testing for allergy and determined I was no longer allergic to it. I sensed that during the treatment, some energy shift had happened to make carrot's energy suitable for my body. I then ate one whole carrot stick and did not have any reaction. I tried some other foods I was known to be allergic to and reacted as before, so I knew my assumption was correct. My allergy to carrot was gone because of my contact with the carrot while undergoing acupuncture. My energy and the carrot's energy were repelling prior to that acupuncture treatment. After the treatment, their energies became compatible — no more repulsion!

The repulsive energy between my body and the carrot was presented as an allergy in me. During the acupuncture treatment, my body probably became a powerful charger and was strong enough to change the adverse charge of the carrot to match my body's charge. This resulted in removing my allergy to the carrot. I continued to treat for other items that I previously could not eat. I tested and treated my husband and my son for many of their respective allergies. In a few weeks, we were no longer allergic to many of the foods that previously made us ill. We could eat and enjoy a variety of foods without getting sick. Later, I extended this to my patients who suffered from a multitude of symptoms that arose from allergies.

My complete recovery and return to health has now been duplicated over and over in thousands of my patients. I am convinced that I have discovered something truly wonderful about the treatment of allergies that does not include strict diets, stringent potions of any kind, or isolation to avoid allergy-producing environmental elements. It is this knowledge, as well as the urgent prompting of thousands of my patients who no longer suffer from allergy symptoms, that convinced me to write this book.

Some case studies featured in Chapter 10 have shown how many people who have undergone these treatments now enjoy good health. I receive countless numbers of NAET stories and encouraging testimonials every day not only from my patients, but from NAET patients from everywhere, expressing their desire to share their stories of achieving good health through NAET with other less fortunate allergic victims of the world. These kindhearted, compassionate people will go to any length to spread the word about NAET, so that other allergy-sufferers will be encouraged to get NAET treatments, and eventually achieve freedom from allergy.

Most of them send touching cover letters along with their testimonials, requesting that I print their testimonials in NAET publications, NAET books, or use their testimonials in any way to spread the word about NAET. Some of them send their full addresses, telephone numbers, and e-mail addresses to print along with publications of their testimonials. I would like to apologize to these kindhearted people that I purposely excluded their full addresses and whereabouts from my publications even though they enclosed signed consents. Their good intentions are appreciated very much. I do not think it is necessary for anyone to communicate with ex-patients before they begin their treatments. NAET is a simple, safe, energy balancing technique. No side effects have noted so far if the treatments are administered correctly. I have given the maximum NAET information permitted to share with non-medical readers in my books (information is in each and every book I have written), so that readers will get the basic knowledge about NAET by reading the books alone. Not only that, I do not want to see these noble-minded, good-hearted people become victims by any means. So, just to protect these patients' safety, I did not completely honor their requests.

I would like to express my apology to all NAET patients again for not being able to print all the testimonials I receive daily since I have access only to limited printing. I make a point to read every letter that comes to my office and I want all of you to know that I really cherish them. Most of your testimonials bring tears of happiness to my eyes. I am very thankful to God for permitting me to live a normal life, and I am also very gratified to know that most of you have received similar opportunities of health and happiness through NAET. If any letter needs my personal reply, I make it a point to respond to it; sometimes, my replies will be delayed for months due to lack of time. But your letters will be answered.

Allergic patients do not have to spend the rest of their lives in fear or in a bubble anymore. Instead, they too can live like other normal persons, provided they get treated for their allergies by doctors well trained in NAET.

In Chapter 9, I have included many testimonials from NAET practitioners and their contact information, so that when patients find a practitioner closer to their home, they may approach them directly without wasting time to search in the web sites, or calling my office for their addresses, etc.

The more extensively I studied the subject of allergies, the more I found it to be a truly fascinating, yet highly complex field. Although food allergies as causes for multiple physiological problems have been gaining acceptance as a separate area of medical study in recent years, they certainly have not been given the recognition they deserve. In fact, knowledge of the field is still quite limited, not only among the general public, but also among those who treat allergies, because of the limited volume of available research.

NAET is a simple technique that involves art and science from various medical disciplines. It can give relief from multitudes of commonly seen health disorders, those that originally started with some allergic reactions. It requires patience on the part of the practitioner as well as the patient because it sometimes takes numerous office visits for optimum recovery, especially recovery from long-term or serious health disorders. that NAET is too simple. These people feel that if the testing and treatment procedures are not made complex, they won't work. The fact is that these people with complex minds are either unable to comprehend and follow the simple instructions, or they have become accustomed to the difficulties inherent in most medical practices.

NAET is simple and so effective that some people can experience immediate relief; most people must be treated for the "Basic 10 or 15 allergen groups" first; but I should warn you that many people need a number of office visits to feel better. During my 20 years of practice, I have seen all variations. Some patients with good immune system have taken three or four NAET treatments and lived happily ever after, whereas some others who have poor immune systems, a long list of sickness in the family tree, and poor general health habits, can take hundreds of NAET treatments to straighten out their lives. Chronic suffering, physical, physiological or mental abuse of any kind can cause tissue damage within the body and body organs. People falling in this group take longer time to recover.

Without knowing what is an allergen and what is not an allergen, we continue to expose ourselves to harmful allergens many times every day. Continuous exposures and re-exposures to various allergens throughout one's daily living can aggravate the condition of the body and organs further. In such people, presence of any allergen can trigger immediate allergic reactions, usually attacking the weak organ first. Then eventually, the other organs will be affected. For example: A person with chronic bronchitis or asthma owns a pair of weak, less efficient, hypersensitive lungs. In this person, lungs are the weak area in the body. Whenever this person comes in contact with an allergen his/her lungs will begin to react immediately, producing symptoms like postnasal drip, mucus production in the throat, cough, sinusitis or asthma (these are the common pathological symptoms of the lungs). To get the asthma or chronic bronchitis or sinusitis under control, one may have to eliminate allergies to many allergens from his/her food and environment. But the good news is this: They too can benefit from NAET even though they may have to take a series of treatments.

Today, many people are becoming chemically and environmentally sensitive. Doctors and patients are equally frustrated. Some of these patients live in a bubble-like environment. When one is chemically and environmentally allergic to almost everything around, that person's brain-software is completely disrupted. It can take two to three years of continuous treatments with NAET to replace all the incorrect information with right message about the environment —two to three sessions per week, before one can come out of the bubble into the real world filled with its assorted pollutants, fumes, chemicals, formaldehydes, pesticides and smog. No short cut treatments will work on them. Again the good news is this: When they complete the needed NAET treatments, they too can live a normal life among normal people, among the assorted pollutants, enjoying the benefits of the scientific advancements of the 21st Century.

In planning this book, at first I thought to aim it toward an audience of students and professionals within the health-care field. However, as I thought about it, I came to understand that good health care depends mainly on the patient. It is just as imperative to inform people about their allergies (known, suspected, or hidden) as it is to educate the health-care professional. If the lay reader can learn to find and identify known, suspected or hidden allergens through Nambudripad's Testing Techniques (NTT), the help will be within reach through NAET (Nambudripad's Allergy Elimination Techniques). Therefore, this book is written for both the health-care professionals and also for lay persons, to acquire an understanding of the allergy process within the body and to gain an understanding of the cause, effect and, now, elimination of allergies.

In this book, I do use some specialized terminology that may give some lay readers a harder time and diminish their reading pleasure and understanding. But, rest assured, technical terms are kept to a minimum.

I would feel gratified, indeed, if the up-to-date material compiled herein were to contribute to my readers achieving, maintaining and enjoying good health; and if, through readers in the healing profession, an even larger number of people were to receive the possible benefits.

In this book I would like to have shared all my NAET experiences of twenty years. But I have discovered that it is not wise to compress everything in one book because the book may be too large, consisting of thousands of pages and readers may get discouraged. Instead, I decided to write many small books, called NAET series or Say Good-bye to... series, each pertaining to different manifestations of allergies. This concept may also help the reader to read just the materials that he/she is interested in, for example, Say Good-bye to Arthritis, or Say Good-bye to Asthma, etc.

You can gain more information on NAET testing and treatment processes by reading my previously published books, "Say Good-bye to Illness", "Say Good-bye to ADD & ADHD," "Say Good-bye to Allergy-related Autism," "Say Good-bye to Children's Allergies," "The NAET Guide Book," and "Living Pain Free with Acupressure (a self-help book to manage your pain)." To further enhance your understanding, you might pursue some of the other relevant books and articles listed in the bibliography at the conclusion of this book.

Stay Allergy-Free and Enjoy Better HEALTH!

Dr. Devi S. Nambudripad,
M.D., D.C., L.Ac., Ph.D. (Acu.)
Buena Park, California
January, 2003

End note:

Some readers requested me to write the details of this rice-meal preparation. Please make sure you are not allergic to any of these ingredients before preparation.

The Special Rice Preparation

The ingredients in the special rice-meal: Dry coriander seeds, dried lemon leaves, lemon rind, black pepper, ginger root, brown sugar, dandelion leaves, turmeric, cumin seeds, rock salt, garlic, cinnamon and dried pomegranate skin. All the above ingredients are made into a fine powder. Finely chopped coriander leaves, coconut oil, clarified butter are used fresh.

Function of the herbs in the body:

Coriander leaves clear the neurotoxins from the brain and nervous system. It strengthen the nervous system. It also clears liver meridian.

Coriander seeds cleanse the sinuses, glands and lymphatic system. It clears the spleen meridian.

Cinnamon, lemon rind and rice cleanse and strengthen the lung meridian.

Pepper strengthens the heart and circulatory systems.

Ginger root strengthens the stomach meridian.

Brown sugar strengthens the spleen meridian.

Dandelion leaves strengthen the liver meridian.

Coconut oil strengthens the gall bladder meridian.

Turmeric and cumin seed have antibacterial properties and can help to clean and strengthen the small intestine meridian.

Rock salt is good for the kidney meridians.

Lemon leaves strengthen the bladder meridian

Pomegranate strengthens the large intestine meridian.

Garlic is a natural antibacterial, anti-parasitic and antioxidant that helps clean toxins from the whole system.

Amount of ingredients:

1 cup uncooked rice

2 tablespoons full of coriander powder

1 teaspoonful of chopped coriander leaves

1 teaspoonful of clarified butter

1 teaspoonful of coconut oil

1 teaspoonful of the powder made from rest of the ingredients together.

Salt to taste.

Preparation: Rinse the rice four times with clean water, cook well in eight cups of water, drain when the rice is cooked well. Add coriander powder, three ounces of water and cook again under slow fire until the water is evaporated completely. Add rest of the ingredients, mix well and cover and keep it for 10 minutes before you serve. I often prepare this rice even now, because I enjoy this spicy, delicious rice that saved my life once!

INTRODUCTION

I t is your *human right* to eat whatever food you like to eat, live in whatever environment you like, wear what ever clothes or cosmetics you want, live with whomever you prefer, and be happy. If you are able to accomplish this, you can say that you are healthy physically, physiologically and psychologically. If you are not able to accomplish this, you have an illness.

People without having first-hand knowledge of NAET might get confused by the above statement.

People get sick everywhere. No one knows the real cause. So every one treats the symptoms that one can see by observing the signs and symptoms of a disorder. So we have symptom-oriented treatments. NAET theory believes that some software problems (a Virus perhaps?) in the brain-computer is the cause of allergies and allergy-related illnesses.

NAET is a way to reprogram one's brain to its original state. NAET is the computer virus treatment to help one's brain to remove the faulty program and replace with correct one.

NAET is not a magic cure for anything. I don't want readers to get any wrong idea by reading my above writing. It is pure hard work. Hard work based on stone-hard Oriental medical theory. If you are not willing to work hard, if you expect a magic bullet to cure all your problems, NAET is not for you. If you are willing to work hard, willing to make changes in your life-style, you can get relief of any allergy-based medical symptoms I have mentioned anywhere in this book or in any other book. I have treated every one of those allergy-based problems successfully with NAET. If they are not allergies or originating from allergies, NAET is not the way to go.

The main application of NAET is to remove the adverse reactions between your body and other substances and thus to provide you with good nutrition, and enhance your natural ability to absorb, assimilate the necessary elements from your food and eliminate the unwanted and toxic materials when they get into your body by any means. NAET advices you to test everything around you for possible allergy before you put it in your mouth or apply on your body or bring it close to your body (electromagnetic field). If you are allergic to every ingredient in your diet, no matter how pure and clean your diet is, you will never find a single healthy day in your life. If you are allergic to your own digestive juices (stomach acid (HCL) and digestive enzymes or base), no matter what simple food you eat, no matter what high quality digestive enzymes you take, you will have indigestion (bloating, flatulence, sensation of heaviness, brain fog, overweight, underweight, heaviness in the head, poor elimination, etc.) everyday of your life. People could be allergic to environments: grasses, weeds, flowers, bees, insects, etc. which are supposed to create clean environment, and if you are allergic to them you could never step out of your room without getting sick. If you are allergic to pesticides (pesticides are loaded with heavy metals, mercury, etc.) and other environmental toxins, again you have to close up and stay in your room. Even if you eat carefully, buy everything from health food stores, statistics have shown that an average person in America consumes 100-150- pounds of pesticides a year.

How can you hide from all these and live? When you get treated with NAET, your body will not react to these allergens anymore. When you get them into your body, body will throw them out through natural elimination process without alerting the immune system. As long as you are allergic to these, your body will alert the immune system every time they come near you. After you replace the faulty program with a new, corrected one by treating and clearing the allergies to nutritious foods and products, you will be able to consume them freely without getting sick.

If you check around, you will realize 95% of the human illnesses originate from some form of allergies. So the real cause of your illness is allergies - caused by a virus in one's brain-computer software. The programming error causes inappropriate responses to every stimuli coming into the body. Many people think mercury, pesticides, environmental toxins, childhood immunizations, vaccinations, etc. cause illnesses like autism, ADHD, dyslexia, irritable bowels, even cancer. In my opinion, people's allergic tendency (programming error) makes them react to these toxins and cause such serious illnesses. After the successful NAET treatment program for these toxins, we are finding reversal of such problems.

Almost all children get vaccinated lately. Some percentage suffer from side effects like autism, ADD, etc. Every child who gets vaccinated does not manifest autism or such dangerous diseases. That is a fact everyone knows. Why does the vaccine affect only a certain percentage of children? Why do other children lead healthy, normal lives? Has anyone thought about this? People who are against vaccination and childhood immunization will not like me saying this. But someone has to say this and make people aware of the truth about allergies and their connections with certain types of allergy-based disorders like autism, in order to prevent autism and many such disorders among children.

One might argue that the children who do not react adversely to the vaccines have good immune system. Yes, I do agree. But how did they get good immune system? Either inherited or they have no allergy to the vaccines. Again the allergy is the underlying cause— Allergy to mercury or the vaccine itself. Many of my young patients who suffer from autism and ADHD get completely normal after treating with NAET for their allergy to vaccines, mercury and other toxins, whereas they were pushed away once by other treating medical practitioners to the corner saying that they are "autistic and of course, there is no cure for autism."

So mercury is not the cause for most autism (at least the ones arising from vaccine), it is a mistaken diagnosis. The actual cause of autism is the child's allergy to mercury. One of the latest research data projected that one out of 200 children are turning autistic in this country. If we do not take this data seriously, in a few years we will have autistic people sitting in high places and ruling the country.

If the doctors and parents learn to use NAET testing techniques (read Chapter 6), we can put an end to this vaccine-related autism and allergy-related autism. Children should be tested for the allergy to vaccines before they get the vaccination, not after they get the reactions and damages. No other testing techniques are designed to do this job. But NAET is. If children are already immunized and suffering the consequences, NAET can treat them and most likely they will become normal once again like many other Children have done in the past in NAET offices. How do I get this message across to people?

NAET stresses the importance on life-style changes. Consuming non-allergic food and drinks, living in a non-allergic environment, using non-allergic chemicals, associating with non allergic people, getting adequate exercise, all this means life-style changes. It means giving up eating junk food, and drinking non-nutritious sodas, giving up refined sugars and alcohol and eating more vegetables, and wholesome nutritious foods.

Some people may get scared of that regimen. But I have news for you. When you complete the NAET treatments successfully — (I stress on this: *complete the treatment successfully*— because I have come to know that some practitioners are not doing NAET properly and they are mixing NAET with other treatments and not getting the expected result from NAET treatments), you stop craving wrong things. Your body will begin craving more meaningful items instead of junk food. Things like fresh vegetables, wholesome foods, etc. If you are a sugar addict before NAET, after completing treatments, you will give up eating sugar and you don't even miss it. That is our experience for the past 20 years. You will become health-oriented naturally.

NAET will guide you to the right direction, will give you an opportunity to work hard and get normal. Most people with allergies live in fear. They are afraid to go out of their comfort zones, they are fearful to travel, or eat at a regular restaurant for fear of reactions. You are advised to eat limited food during the treatment phase, but after the 25-hours of each treatment, you should eat non-allergic, wholesome food to receive adequate nutrition. After successful completion of allergy treatment you don't react much to the foods and environments. Once in a while if you ate at McDonald's or Taco Bell, your body will not collapse. You will be able to handle it with ease. That is the 21st Century treatment. You will be free to live in this world again. Eating refined foods and junk food can put more stress on your system without giving you any benefit of nutrients. You need to live sensibly. Moderation of everything at every level is the key to long-term good health.

Say Good-bye to Your Allergies will help you understand your illness and will assist you in finding the right help to achieve better health.

Say Good-bye to Your Allergies will show you how certain commonly used products can cause health problems; how such problems have a domino effect that can end in serious complications; how your problems can relate to allergy, a traditionally under-diagnosed or misdiagnosed condition; and, how allergies can manifest into myriad symptoms that might seem unrelated.

It's not enough to treat symptoms with medication or a piece-meal therapy. These usually just put a "bandage" on the sore, so to speak. *Say Good-bye to Your Allergies* gets to the root of health problems and will help you in eliminating their causes.

With this book you can now learn how to reprogram your brain (central nervous system) to accept all foods, substances, products, and environments as neutral or beneficial. Not all in one session. You may need many sessions with your practitioner or do it yourself if you have many mild or hidden allergies. You will learn how allergy might have caused your health problems. You will learn how genetic allergies and allergy-related illness can now be controlled.

Your brain is an obliging organ that has been searching for ways to help you feel better through much trial and error and various levels of homeostasis (balance). Now it can do the job it has been trying to do. Through NAET, your reprogrammed brain will have learned to accept substances it previously rejected and will allow your body to react normally to the elements of your life so you can get on your way to perfect health.

NAET is developed by Dr. Devi S. Nambudripad, who has been treating patients with this technique since 1983, and teaching other health professionals how to administer it since 1989. To date, more than 7,000 licensed medical practitioners have been trained in NAET procedures and are practicing all over the world. For more information on NAET or for an NAET practitioner near you, log on to the NAET website: www.naet.com.

How Do I Know I Have Allergies?

If you experience any unusual physical, physiological or emotional symptoms without any obvious reason, you can suspect an allergy.

Who Should Use This Book?

Anyone who is suffering from food and environmental allergies or anyone suffering from an allergy-related disease or condition should read this book. This natural, non invasive technique is ideal to treat infants, children, grown-ups, old and debilitated people who suffer from mild to severe allergic reactions without altering their current plan of treatment. NAET encourages the use all medications, supplements or other therapies while going through the

NAET program. When the patient gets better, the patient's regular physician can reduce or alter the dosage of drugs.

How is This Book Organized?

Chapter 1: Explains allergies in general term.

Chapter 2: Describes NAET.

Chapter 3: Describes the categories of allergies and allergens.

Chapter 4: Explains Nambudripad's Testing Techniques and gives you information on various other allergy testing techniques.

Chapter 5: Explains the abnormal functions of the meridians when there is energy disturbance in them.

Chapter 6: Explains Muscle Response Testing (MRT) to detect allergies, the main testing technique used in NAET testing procedures.

Chapter 7: Discusses NAET allergen samples.

Chapter 8: Describes a few NAET self-treatment techniques.

Chapter 9: NAET practitioners share their NAET experiences.

Chapter 10: NAET patients share their NAET results.

Glossary: This section will help you to understand the appropriate meaning of the medical terminology used in this book.

Resources: Provided to assist you in finding natural products and consultants to support you while you work with your allergies.

Bibliography: Since NAET is an energy balancing treatment, supporting bibliography on this subject is hard to find. This book cannot be completed without mentioning valuable information on Oriental Medicine and acupuncture, because NAET has developed from Oriental Medicine. Since NAET uses basic information from allopathy, kinesiology and chiropractic, books explaining these subject are also given in the bibliography.

Index: A detailed index is included to help you quickly and easily locate your area of interest.

CHAPTER 1

What is an Allergy

A n allergy can be defined as an "overreaction" or "hyper sensitivity" of the body's immune system to certain substances. According to Oriental medical theory, allergies and allergy-based disorders are the results of long-term energy disturbances in the energy pathways (please read Chapter ten, Acupuncture Meridians in Say Good-bye to Illness by me or in any acupuncture text books given in Bibliography). Severe allergic reactions are caused by severe energy disturbance in one or more energy meridians.

Causes of allergies

Disruption of the software program of the brain: The main cause of allergies is the computer software error in one's brain-computer or let's say one's brain-computer software has a 'Virus.' This virus causes malfunction of the software, in turn all body functions are disrupted. This causes the body to be sensitive to everything around the body. The malfunctioning program does not recognize things around the body anymore. This software virus may have found its way into the body through the following routes:

- Heredity: An allergic tendency is inherited from parents

and family as dominant or recessive, but allergic manifestation may vary from generation to generation. For example, if a parent suffered from migraines, offspring may suffer from eczema or asthma and not necessarily have migraines.

• Toxins: From food, drinks, medicines, herbs, vitamins, environments, animal epithelial, animal dander, pesticides, lead, mercury, dry cleaning chemicals, house cleaning chemicals, chemically treated city water, drinking water, industrial waste, polluted air, pollen, smoke, cigarette smoke, etc.

• Infections: Toxins produced in the body from invasions of microorganisms such as virus, bacteria, parasite, yeast, candida, ticks (lyme disease), etc.

• Vaccinations and immunizations/ toxins

• A depressed immune system: Chronic illnesses, autoimmune disorders, etc.

• Malabsorption disorders: Nutritional deficiencies, digestive problems, poor absorption and assimilation of nutrients due to an allergy to the nutrients, eating overcooked, infected, or unsuitable food or unavailability of food.

• Hormonal deficiencies: Removal of reproductive organs, dysfunction of ovaries, thyroid glands, hypothalamus, deficiency of female and male hormones, adrenals and pituitary hormones

• Post-traumatic disorders: Surgery, accidents, delivery, stressful work, school, life-style, war veterans, etc.

• Radiation and geopathic stress: Working long hours with computers, sitting in front of television sets, living near or under powerful electrical cables, living near power plants, exposure to radioactive materials, working under extreme weather conditions without proper clothing.

• Poor Physical Activities

• Emotional traumas: Disharmony of mind-body-spirit due to traumas from past or present, childhood abuses, abuses and traumas in other ages, troubled emotions like chronic fear, anger, cult association, victimization, etc.

In people with allergies, the normal imprint (memory) about the harmlessness of substances such as peanut, fish, pollen, dust, perfume, etc., has somehow been erased from the brain's memory during the genetic transference or during certain stresses of life (exposure to extreme radiation, bacterial or chemical toxins, etc.) and has substituted the memory with new information that identifies the substance as being dangerous. Thus, the immune system mistakes a harmless substance for a dangerous intruder it must destroy. When a person with allergies is exposed to something it perceives to be an allergen, the immune system produces antibodies to fight it as a harmful invader.

Allergies usually first appear in infancy or childhood. However, onset of symptoms can occur at any age or, in some cases, reappear after many years of inactivity. An allergy is generally a hereditary condition. An allergic tendency is inherited, but it may manifest totally differently than that of one's ancestors. The age of onset of an allergic condition depends on the degree of inheritance. The stronger the genetic factor, the earlier in life is the onset. Studies have shown that when both parents were (or are) allergy-sensitive, 75 to 100 percent of their offspring react to the same or similar allergens. When neither of the parents is (or was) sensitive to allergens, the probability of producing allergic offspring drops dramatically, to less than ten percent.

According to statistics released by the CDC (Center for Disease Control), more than 50 million Americans suffer from allergic diseases every year. Up to two million, or 8 percent, of children in the United States estimated to be affected by food allergy. Up to 2 percent of adults are so affected. According to the CDC (1996 statistics), chronic sinusitis is the most commonly reported chronic respiratory tract disease, affecting 12.6 percent of people (approximately 38 million). According to the Journal of the American Medical Association (270:2456-63, 1993), allergy to the venom of stinging insects (honeybees, wasps, hornets, yellow jackets, and fire ants) is relatively common, with prevalence of systemic reactions in American adults of 3.3 percent. The Journal of Allergy and Clinical Immunology (103:559-62, 1999) reported that peanut allergies affect approximately 3 million Americans and cause the most severe food-induced allergic reactions. AAAAI (the American College of Allergy, Asthma and Immunology) reported that seasonal allergic rhinitis, often referred to as "hay fever," affects more than 35 million people in the United States. According to a statistical report from AAAAI noted that if one parent has allergic disease, the estimated risk of a child developing allergies is 48 percent; the child's estimated risk grows to 70 percent if both parents have a history of allergy.

People suffer from allergic manifestation in varying degrees because of difference in parental inheritance. But regardless of age, gender, race, or inheritance, anyone can manifest allergies at any time if the tendency is present.

In some cases, even when parents had no allergies, their offspring might carry the genetic possibility for allergy. In these cases, various possibilities exist:

• Parents may have suffered from a serious disease or condition. Example: Malaria contracted before the child was born and caused alteration in the genetic codes.

• Expectant mother may have been exposed to harmful substances like radiation (X-ray), chemicals, too much caffeine, alcohol, drugs or antibiotics.

• Toxins could have caused genetic mutation as the result of a disease (streptococcal infection as in strep-throat, measles or chicken pox).

• A woman may have suffered severe emotional trauma(s): Abuse, divorce, abandonment, death of the spouse, etc. during pregnancy

• Parents may have suffered severe malnutrition (not getting enough food, or not assimilating due to poor absorption due to allergies), possibly causing the growing embryo to undergo cell mutation.

Any of these may have caused alteration of the genetic codes and altered messages to be carried over to the next generation. The result: The organs and tissues that are supposed to develop normally may have impaired function.

People can be allergic to anything they come in contact with. If one begins to check around — even with so-called healthy people — one will find obvious or hidden allergens as a causative factor in almost all health problems. These allergens may include:

- Animals and animal products: Animal epithelial, animal dander, wool, lanolin, etc.

- Biohazard agents: Industrial waste, insecticides and pesticides

- Bed material: Mattress, pillow and linen

- Building materials: Paint, paint thinner, insulation, dry wall, formaldehyde and ceramic tiles

- Cosmetics: Body lotion, make-up, lipstick and hair products

- Drinks: Water, alcohol, soft drinks, coffee and tea

- Dust Particles: House dust, industrial dust

- Fabrics: Polyester and other petrochemical-based fabrics, but also nylon, cotton, silk, rayon, etc.

- Flowers: Perfume from the flowers, etc.

- Food: Regular and genetically engineered vegetables, legumes and fruits

- Food additives: Sulfites, nitrates, M.S.G., food colorings

- Gasoline and other crude oil products

- Environmental: Grass, weeds, trees, pollens, flowers,

sand

- Herbs and herb products: Tea, supplements
- Insect venom: Bee stings, scorpion and mosquitoes
- Latex: Rubber, elastics, rubber backing or sole of the shoes
- Lead: Lead piping, lead pencils, paint and heavy metals
- Medications: Prescription or over-the-counter
- Mercury: Dental amalgam, fish, pesticides, and antibacterial agents
- Microorganisms: Bacteria, viruses, parasites, mycoplasma and chlamydia,
- Mold: Yeast, fungi, candida
- Nutritional Supplements: Vitamins, minerals
- Paper products: Newspaper, toilet paper, books, etc.
- Perfume: Cologne, after-shave lotion, soap
- Plastics: Computer keyboard, mouse and household products
- Schoolwork materials
- Foot wear: Shoes, socks, slippers
- Tools: Working materials
- Vinyl: Shoes, slippers, handbags, sofa, curtains, vertical and mini blinds, etc.
- Weather conditions like cold, snow, heat, humidity, wind
- Wood: Furniture, cabinet, tables, pencil and decorations

In sensitive individuals, contact with any allergen can produce a variety of symptoms, in varying degrees ranging from mild itching to severe swelling of the tissues, or mild fatigue to severe anaphylaxis. The ingested, inhaled or contacted allergens are capable of alerting the body's immune system. The frightened and confused immune system then commands the production and immediate release of immunoglobulins and other chemical mediators.

These immune system mediators are released as part of the body's immune response to counteract the effect of the invading foreign substances (allergens). Some people may be allergic to their own immune system mediators. In these sensitive people, their endogenous secretions or their immune system mediators produce abnormal physical, physiological and psychological symptoms in varying degrees when these chemicals are released into the bloodstream to fight what the body considers dangerous invaders. When the body reacts adversely to the immune mediators, the body loses the fight to the invader. Then the weak body exaggerates the physical, physiological or psychological response toward the invader, which then causes disease.

There are millions of potential allergens. Our bodies interact and react with them hundreds of times every day. Only some people react adversely where others live happily among them, eating and enjoying their benefits. These normal people have normal immune systems. When the immune system is working properly, allergic reactions are kept under control. A normal body releases appropriate immune system mediators to fight the invader and win. These mediators bring the situation under control in seconds by enhancing body functions to speed up the metabolic functions: Neutralize the toxin or enhance the digestion in case the attacker is a food-protein, as in peanut; neutralize the chemical reaction in case the invader is pesticide, mercury, or a swimming pool chemical; destroy the toxin in case the attacker is bacteria, virus, or a parasite, etc.

Immune system also releases chemicals like histamine, endorphin, enkephalin, leukotrien, bradykinin, interleukin, etc., which may cause symptoms such as inflammation of the mucous membranes of the nose and airways, or inflammation elsewhere in the body, in the pretext of neutralizing or throwing out the invader. In sensitive individuals, these mediators may also cause increased or decreased: Heart rates, body temperature, blood pressure, blood circulation, mucus production, sweat production, urine production, muscle contraction, muscle relaxation, breathing difficulty, choking sensation, even an anaphylactic shock.

What began as an innocent case of mistaken identity is now an allergic reaction, possibly causing death if there is a complete shutdown of the system.

For those whose lives are merely disrupted by the discomfort of the allergic reaction, traditional treatments with simple antihistamine or topical remedies can bring relief. But for more serious sufferers, either long-term immunotherapy or complete avoidance is the only hope traditional medicine has generally been able to offer. Immunotherapy, of course, is expensive and time-consuming, and it often does not present a satisfactory outcome. Most people finally resort to a lifetime of depriving themselves of the many things in life that would otherwise bring them joy and fulfillment. Common complaints are, "My allergies have taken control of my life," and, "The very things that I want to make me happy are the very things that I react to the most."

Even with avoidance, there is no guarantee that allergy sufferers will be able to stay away from every situation and still remain reaction free. With the progress of science and technology, our modern life-styles have changed dramatically. New products, which are potential allergens for many people are being developed every day. The quality of life has improved but for some allergic people, scientific achievements have merely created more nightmares.

In order to enjoy life, the allergic patient must find ways to overcome adverse reactions to chemicals and other allergens produced by technology. Nambudripad's Allergy Elimination Techniques program (NAET) offers the prospect of relief to those who suffer from constant allergic reactions by reprogramming the brain to better health. Just like rebooting a computer, we can reboot our nervous system through NAET to overcome adverse reactions of brain or body or both.

Many symptoms of different diseases overlap with symptoms of allergies. It is because we live in a symptom-oriented society. As soon as a person manifests a particular symptom(s), we give a medical name. Then onwards, we recognize that symptom by a specific name. For example: A man drinks a glass of orange juice every morning with his breakfast. He feels tingling and numbness on both feet below ankles by 10:00 am. His condition is named "neuropathy" due to unknown origin. We have various treatments and medications available to reduce or eliminate the symptoms as soon as they manifest. Most of the time the treatments will work. The symptoms diminishes or disappears instantly when the patient takes the pills; doctors and patients are happy and they do not think about the symptoms anymore until it returns at another time. No one seems to take time to look into the cause that produced the symptom initially as long as it responded to the treatment. Such was the case of Marion, 62, who suffered from neuropathy for 9 years. After suffering from an ideopathic neuropathy in his feet for years, he was tested by an NAET practitioner and found that he was allergic to vitamin C and citrus mix. When he was treated for the allergy to vitamin C (orange juice) with NAET, his ideopathic neuropathy disappeared and has not returned in five years. Tania 42, suffered from headaches over the eyes and forehead at about 5pm. daily for the past 7 years. When she reported this to her physician, he advised her to take an Exedrin PM daily at the start of her headache. Without fail she took one Exedrin PM. daily at 5:00 pm. She received freedom from her headache in ten minutes after taking the pill. Next day again her headache would return. She never left home without Exedrin PM.

When she came to me, I evaluated her condition. I took a detailed history about her eating and drinking habits and found out that daily, about 4:30 PM she had a cup of tea regularly. She never missed that tea. She never drank tea or coffee at any other time during the day. She never liked chocolate and took no other products with caffeine. She was found to be allergic to tea that was affecting her Stomach meridian that produced the frontal headache. She was treated for tea with NAET. Next evening she did not drink tea since she had to avoid tea for 25 hours and she did not get a headache. First time in years she didn't take the Exedrin PM. Next day onwards she drank her regular tea but never got another 5:00 pm headache.

A Self-Evaluation

Do you suffer from any allergy? or Allergy-related disorder? Below is an allergy-check list to help you evaluate yourself to see if you have any active or hidden allergies.

A sensible solution can be found if you can identify the source of your problem.

Please describe your chief problem in one sentence.

_____

_____

When did your problem begin? Please write approximate date and time if **you don't remember the exact date, time and event.**_____

Rate your symptoms on the following list on a 0-10 scale

1. How is your energy generally at these following hours?

6 am [ ], 8 am [ ], 10 am [ ], 12 noon [ ], 2 pm [ ], 4 pm [ ],
6 pm [ ], 6 pm [ ], 8 pm [ ], 10 pm [ ],12 am [ ], 2 am [ ],4 am [ ]

2. How is your appetite?————————— [   ]

3. How is your digestion? —————————[   ]

4. How is your elimination? —————————[   ]

5. How is your sleep? ————————— [   ]

6. How is your mental clarity? ————— [   ]

7. How is your general well-being?   — [   ]

Organ-Meridian Association Clock

It takes two hours to circulate energy through one energy meridian. If the energy can travel through the meridians without any obstruction in the flow, one should feel the overall energy very high. If there is any energy disturbance in the meridian, it will reflect on one's health by feeling fatigued or poor energy. Check your energy level every two even hours when the energy is in the center of each meridian: Check at 6:00 am to find out the status of Large Intestine meridian, etc. (5-7 am is the meridian time for LI). After you find your weak time find the corresponding meridian (s) from the list below. Then go to Chapter 5 in this book (detail information about the acupuncture meridians is given in Chapter 10 in Say Good-bye to Illness) to find out more about your health. Then go to Chapter 8 to learn the self-balancing techniques. Do it once or twice a day for a few weeks. No matter what condition you are in, your energy will get better.

Names of the Meridians

Lung (Lu) - 3-5 am

Large Intestine (LI) - 5-7 am

Stomach (St) - - 7-9 am

Spleen (Sp) - 9-11 am

Heart - 11-1 pm

Small Intestine - (SI) - 1-3 pm

Urinary Bladder (UB) - 3-5 p.m.

Kidney (Ki) - 5-7 pm

Pericardium (PC or CI) -7-9 pm

Triple warmer (TW) - 9-11 -pm

Gall Bladder (GB) - 11-1 am

Liver (Lv) - 1-3 am

ORGAN CLOCK
INDICATING TIMES OF GREATEST ACTIVITY

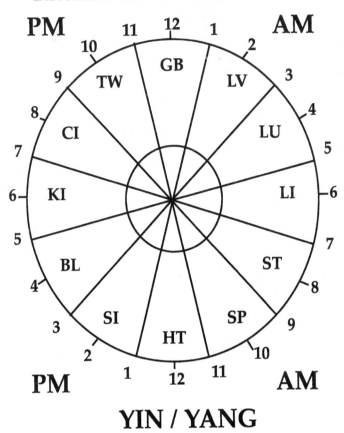

Figure 1-7
Organ-Meridian Association Time

Allergy Sympom Checklist

Please read the following list of symptoms in the next few pages. They could be caused from allergies. Many thousands of people have received relief from these symptoms by treating with NAET. Please rate your symptoms on a scale of 0- 5: (0= no symptoms; 1= mild symptoms; 2= moderate symptoms; 3= severe symptoms; 4= extremely-severe; 5=near death).

—Acne

—Addiction to alcohol

—Addiction to caffeine,

—Addiction to chocolate

—Addiction to coffee

— Addiction to drugs

— Addiction to food

— Addiction to smoking

— Addiction to sugar

— Addictions to carbohydrate

—Aggression

— Allergy to animals

— Allergy to aspirin

— Allergy to bee stings

— Allergy to cold

— Allergy to corn

— Allergy to fish

— Allergy to food additives

— Allergy to food colorings

— Allergy to gasoline

— Allergy to hair dye

— Allergy to heat

— Allergy to humidity

— Allergy to insects

— Allergy to latex

—Allergy to mercury

—Allergy to milk products

—Allergy to mushroom

—Allergy to mold

—Allergy to newspaper ink

—Allergy to nuts

—Allergy to paper

—Allergy to peanuts

—Allergy to penicillin

—Allergy to perfume

—Allergy to plastics

—Allergy to pollens

—Allergy to proteins

—Allergy to radiation

—Allergy to razer blade

—Allergy to salt

—Allergy to shellfish

—Allergy to smells
—Allergy to sugar
—Allergy to trees
—Allergy to weeds
—Allergy to wheat/gluten
—Amnesia, temporary
—Anemia
—Angina-like pains
—Anxiety attacks
—Arthritis
—Asthma, bronchial
—Asthma, cardiac
—Athletes foot
—Attention deficit disorder
— Backache
—Bone pains
— Bipolar disorders
— Biting nails.
— Bladder problems
— Blurred vision at night
—Bowel disorder
— Brain fog
—Breast-pain
—Breast-lumps
—Breast-swelling
— Burning feet
— Burning in the groin
— Burning on urination

— Burning urine
— Candida/yeast
—Canker sores
— Cannot be pacified
— Cardiac arrhythmias
— Cervical dysplacia
— Chemical sensitivities
— Chronic cough
—Chronic fatigue
—Chronic low grade fever
—Chronic nasal congestion
—Clumsiness
—Cold extremities
—Cold intolerance
—Cold sores
—Colitis
—Compulsive behavior
—Constipation
—Cough
—Craving fat
—Craving spices
—Craving salt
—Craving sour
—Craving sweets
—Craving bitters
—Craving onions
— Crohns' disease
—Cunjunctivitis

—Cuts heal slowly

—Dandruff

—Decreased sex drive

—Dermatitis

—Depression

—Destructive

—Diabetes

—Diarrhea

—Difficulty in walking

—Difficulty in swallowing

—Distractibility

—Diverticulitis

—Dizziness

—Double vision

—Dream disturbed sleep

—Dry eyes

—Dry mouth

—Dry skin

—Dryness

—Dyslexia

—Ear aches

—Ear infections

— Eating dirt

—Eating disorders

—Eczema

—Edema of the feet

—Elbow pain

—Eyelids puffy

—Emphysema

—Enuresis (bed wetting)

— Erratic disruptive behavior

— Excessive appetite

— Excessive drooling

— Excessive flatulence

— Excessive salivation

— Excessive sweating

— Exercise-induced asthma

— Failing memory

— Fainting spells

— Fatigue

— Fear

— Fever of unknown origin

— Feels insecure

— Fibromyalgia

— Fibrocystic breast

— Food cravings

— Food sensitivity

—Forgetfulness

— Formaldehyde allergy

— Frequent repetitive activity

— Frequent bronchitis

— Frequent ear infection

— Frequent flu's and colds.

— Frequent infections

— Frequent pneumonia

— Frequent sore throat

— Frequent sweating

— Frequent urination

—Gags easily

—Gallstones

— Gastric distress

— Gastric ulcer

— General body aches

— General fatigue

— General itching

— Glaucoma

—Greasy food upsets

— Groin pain

— Growing pains

— Hair colorings

—Hay-fever

—Hair loss

— Hair pulling

— Halitosis

—Hand flicking

—Head banging

—Headache/afternoon

—Headache/migraine

—Headache over the eyes

—Headaches/sinus

—Headache/morning

—Headaches under the eyes

—Hearing loss/decreased

—Heartburn

—Heart irregularities

—Hemorrhoids

—Herpes-1

—Herpes-2

—Hepatitis

—High altitude problem

—High blood pressure

—High cholesterol

—Hives

—Hoarseness

—Holds on to people and objects.

—Hot flashes

—Hungry between meals

—Hyperactivity

—Hypoglycemia

—Impaired ability to role-play

—Impaired speech

—Impaired peer relationships

—Impulsivity

—Increased sex drive

—Increased thirst

—Indigestion

—Infertility

—Internal tremor

—Insomnia

—Irregular periods

—Irritability

—Irritable bowels

—Itchy eyes

—Jock itch

—Joint pains

—Keyed up, fails to calm

—Knee pains

—Labored breathing

—Leaky gut syndrome

—Learning disabilities

—Light sensitivity

—Listlessness

—Loss of taste

—Loose stools

—Loud talk

—Low backache

—Low blood pressure

—Low body temperature

—Low libido

—Lump in the breast

—Lump in the throat

—Lupus

—Lymph node tenderness

—Metallic taste in the mouth

—Mid backache

—Migrating pains

—Milk causes discomfort

—Mood swings

—Mucus in the throat

—Multiple sclerosis

—Muscle cramps at night

—Muscle pain

—Muscle spasms

—Nasal polyps

—Nausea

—Neck pains

—Nervous stomach

—Neuralgia

—Night sweats

—Nose-bleed

—Neuropathies

—Numbness anywhere in the body

—Obsessive behavior

—Ovarian cyst

—Pain between shoulders

—Pain on the heels

—Pain anywhere in the body without reason

—Panic attacks

—Paranoia

—Parasitic infestation

—Parrot-like talking

—Phobias

—Picking at skin.

—PMS

—Poor appetite

—Poor concentration

—Poor memory

—Post nasal drip

—Premature graying

—Prone to infections

—Prostate troubles

—Psoriasis

—Recurrent prostatitis
—Red blood cells low
—Red blood cells high
—Red eyes
—Repeated dental infection
—Restless leg syndrome
—Reflex sympathetic dystrophy
—Ring worm
—Ringing in the ears
—Sadness
—Sand-like feeling in the eyes
—Sciatic neuralgia
—Scleroderma
—Seizures
—Sensitive to cold
—Sensitive to heat
—Shoulder pain
—Short term memory loss
—Shortness of breath
—Sighs frequently
—Sinusitis
—Skin peels
—Skin problems
—Sleep apnea
—Sleepy during the day
—Slow pulse
—Slow starter
—Smell-decreased

—Sneezing attacks
—Sore throat
—Startles easily
—Strokes
—Strong lights irritates
—Swollen joints, ankles
—Thickening skin
—Thinning skin
—Throat constriction
—Thyroid problem
—Tightness in the chest
—Tingling around the mouth
—Tingling anywhere in the body
—Tourette's syndrome
—Tires too easily
—Toxicity to heavy metal
—Toxicity to pesticides
—Ulcerative colitis
—Uncontrollable body move ments
— Unable to fall asleep at night
—Unable to go back to sleep upon wakening
—Unable to sleep for long hours without waking
—Unexplained chest pain
—Unexplained pain in the body
—Unreasonable anger
—Unrefreshing sleep

—Unusual weight loss

—Upper backaches

—Urinary tract disorder

—Urination difficult

—Urine amount decreased

—Urine amount increased

—Uterine polyp

—Vaginal discharge

—Varicose veins

—Vomiting frequently

—Vulvodynia

—Vertigo

—Warts

—Weak nails

—Wake up during the night

—Watery eyes

—Weight gain for no reason

—Weight loss

—White blood cells low

—White blood cells high

—White spots

—Worrier

—Yeast infections

—Other

What is Your Score?

If you have all zero's you are very healthy.

If you have more **'1'**, you have hidden allergies. Your symptoms are not manifesting yet. If you get into a stressful situation, or if your immune system gets stressed out they may begin to bother you or you may genetically transfer your allergic tendencies to your children or grandchildren. If you could treat the NAET Basics, probably your allergies may never manifest into symptoms or transfer to your children.

If you have more **'2'** and no **'3', '4' or '5'**: You have very mild symptoms. Please find a practitioner and get the Basics treated. or use self-help treatments to eliminate some of your allergies. Please read Chapter 8 for more information on self-treatments.

If you have scored **'3'** and **'4'** in more than **10** areas, you should make an appointment to have a complete checkup by a qualified doctor, and see an NAET practitioner as soon as possible to get your Basics treated with NAET.

If you have scored all **'5'** you could be in serious condition. I would suggest that you see your family doctor immediately, check into a hospital, have all the tests done, have the hospital feed you some nutritious drinks by mouth or intravenous. After you stabilize your present condition, find an NAET practitioner and begin treatments starting from the basics. It is never too late to get treated with NAET. Before you know you may be enjoying best health like everyone else.

CHAPTER 2

What is NAET?

Nambudripad's Allergy Elimination Technique (NAET) is a natural, painless, and non-invasive treatment used to permanently eliminate food and environmental allergies. This treatment does not involve the use of drugs, herbs, vitamins, or other supplements. However, NAET may be used in conjunction with other forms of treatments and therapies including drugs, herbs, vitamins, minerals, enzymes and other supplements, if found appropriate to improve or enhance one's health. Each item, however, should be tested and cleared for any possible allergy before using.

NAET utilizes a combination of kinesiology, acupuncture/acupressure, nutritional management and a specific type of spinal manipulative procedure from chiropractic to accomplish allergy elimination.

NAET uses standard medical diagnostic procedures and standard allergy testing procedures from kinesiology and chiropractic (read Chapter 4) and an electrodermal computerized allergy testing procedure to detect an allergy. These above testing modalities are used initially to identify the problem. After detecting the allergies, NAET uses a simple kinesiological muscle response testing (MRT) on a daily basis to evaluate the response of the patient to the treatment.

If used properly, MRT has the unique ability to retrieve information from one's autonomic nervous system about most stages of one's health problems (mild, moderate or severe symptoms).

NAET also utilizes Oriental medical principles to evaluate the health status of a person by detecting energy blockages in acupuncture meridians.

NAET evaluates the status of the compatibility of daily consumed food, drinks, supplements to trace the cause of the pain and discomforts experienced on a daily basis. NAET emphasizes right nutrition to get the best result, whatever one's problem may be. You are what you eat! The secret to good health is achieved through correct nutrition. What is correct nutrition? Correct or Right nutrition does not mean buying expensive food, drinks or supplements. It means non-allergic food, drinks and supplements.

Around mid-400 B.C., nearly 2500 years ago, Hippocrates, a Greek physician whom we call the "Father of Medicine," noted that cheese caused severe reactions in some people, while others could eat and enjoy it with no unpleasant after-effects. Three hundred years later, the Roman philosopher, Lucretius said, "What is food for some may be fierce poison for others." From this observation has come our expression, "One man's meat is another man's poison."

"A doctor should begin with simple treatments, trying to cure by diet before he administers drugs. No illness that can be treated by diet should be treated by any other means." Hippocrates wrote this in 460 - 377BC. He also expressed more wisdom on diet and nutrition, "If we could give every individual the right amount of nourishment and exercise, not too little and not too much, we would have found the safest way to health." I emphatically believe in his powerful statements about nutrition. But I do not think he could foresee the depth of nutritional involvement with numerous allergic disorders we see today among our population.

Confirmation of diagnosis is achieved through standard medical diagnostic procedures and by various laboratory procedures.

The actual allergy elimination treatments utilize non-force chiropractic, spinal manipulative procedures, and mild acupressure (or acupuncture) treatments on specific points in the body. These reflex and acupuncture points are situated at various bodily locations that relate to the acupuncture meridians. After treatment, to achieve best results with NAET, a person should avoid any contact with the treated allergen for 24-25 hours.

Some confused, misinformed healthcare professionals who have observed certain positive changes in their patients' health condition with NAET treatments received elsewhere, but not had any first-hand knowledge about NAET, often confuse their patients by telling them, "NAET is like turning off a fire alarm when the fire is burning and just letting the fire continue to burn inside." In fact the opposite is true with NAET. It programs the brain to turn on the built-in sprinkler system at the very first sign of any smoke. After the successful completion of NAET treatments, the smoke never progresses into a fire and the fire alarm never has to turn on again. I wish this doubting Thomas-group could come forward and learn the true art of NAET so that they themselves and their patients could benefit from their learning and incorporate their learning into their practices.

I was treated for my allergies two decades ago and none of the treated allergens ever bothered me again. According to our existing knowledge on allergies, experts believe that allergies in remission may reappear after some years of inactivity. I would not disagree with their expertise, but I still think "20 years" is a good long time to live in anticipation. After 20 years of healthy life, if my allergies decide to reappear, I will not complain about it at all; I would be happy to go through the treatments all over. But I am still waiting for the reappearance of my treated allergies if they would ever return.

Many scientifically oriented people ask me, why have I not published all my discoveries and the actual clinical studies in medical journals yet? As soon as some one discovers something in medical field, they immediately rush to publish it before they share it with anyone to secure their position in the world for the simple fear that someone might steal it and put it under their name. I do not worry about such things. As soon as I discover something, I have to tell everyone about it the very next day. I will begin checking and treating all my patients immediately using my new ideas. I will also inform all my students, NAET practitioners right away. Am I not concerned about someone else stealing my discovery and labeling with someone else's name?

In fact that has already happened many times. Many of my students have rediscovered what I have discovered 20 years ago, called it something else and presented to the world as their own discovery. But I believe, duplication is the highest form of flattery. When I discovered NAET, I was ecstatic, and happy beyond any word can express my feelings. Some good friends advised me not to share my discovery with others until I did some studies and publish them in the medical journals. I did some placebo controlled double blind studies to prove it to myself that I wasn't dreaming about the results and it can be duplicated in others. I did not publish the studies. Instead I began training more practitioners in NAET.

NAET gave me a new lease on my life. I know there are many millions suffering now, like the way I did once. My real mission in life is to bring NAET to all the needy people all over the world—if someone stole my technique and presented to others, he/she is still indirectly helping my mission. As long as people get benefit from NAET in any form, I am happy.

The main reason I didn't show much urgency in publishing my discovery because, I was anticipating my allergies to return. I wasn't sure how long NAET treatments lasted since I am the originator and I did not have any place to look for answers to my puzzling questions. I wanted to be sure before I published any data. Time was the only judge. So I decided to wait for 20 years before I believed in it fully. Now I have reached at the 20-year mark, I have come to believe that NAET is in fact able to cure allergies permanently. The health records of my own allergy treatment history of 20 years, my family's record and my pioneer patients' records have proven that to me.

Now our office has launched into many researches. Various clinical trials, double-blind studies, short and long-term studies are under way on different age groups, on various allergy-based pain disorders, and on other aspects of illnesses.

The Development of NAET

My own severe health problems propelled me into extensive study of allergy and allergy-related illnesses (see preface). During my education and early practice as an allergist, while using eclectic methods of allergy treatments, I discovered this technique that eliminated most of my health problems. I began conducting research in 1983 about my new discovery, with the goal of solving my health problems that had plagued me since my birth in India. Eventually, my intense search resulted in the development of this new, effective approach for detection and elimination of allergies and allergy-related health disorders of all types.

While working on my Ph.D. at Samra University of Oriental Medicine in Los Angeles, I observed that people presenting allergic symptoms often responded favorably to acupuncture or acupressure treatments. Education in Oriental medicine helped me to realize the systemic relationship between contact with an allergen and the resulting neurophysiological effects produced in the body. I felt that if one can clearly understand the entry of the invader into the body, it should be easy to remove it. Acupuncture and Oriental medical training helped me to understand the exact mechanism of entry of the invader into one's body. I decided to focus my attention on reversing the invader's journey. I was desperate to put an end to my allergic reactions and health problems and I believed that if I focused my innate energy into getting well, I could be well.

Then one day, the solution happened totally unexpectedly! Just the way I had been dreaming all along. The solution was NAET— stimulating the various acupuncture points in a specific pattern I was able to overcome my extreme allergic reactions to various foods. I named this treatment NAET— Nambudripad's Allergy Elimination Techniques. There was nothing new in this treatment that was not in practice already. Chiropractors manipulated the spine and people found health for many years. Acupuncturists needled the same areas where chiropractors worked on and achieved similar results. Nutritionists achieved great results on their patients by manipulating their nutrients. As I studied each system, I was convinced that all health professionals, even though they all approached slightly differently, depending on their educational background, were unanimously working for the same goal—to get their patient well. Since I was educated in all these areas I was familiar with all these wonderful techniques. I applied all these techniques and information together to get me well, in that attempt, generated totally a different procedure and achieved great results — permanent elimination of dangerous allergies. It was very exciting!

We have done a few studies (double blind studies, clinical trials, and comparison studies) to observe the effectiveness of NAET on various allergies and allergy-related disorders. For various reasons, we have not published them yet. We will be doing them in the near future.

Here is a glimpse into some of our unpublished studies.

Unpublished Studies

Title: Effects of NAET as Relates to 15 of the Most
            Common Subjective Patient Complaints.

Objective: To determine the average number of office visits
            (Allergy elimination treatments), using <u>NAET</u>
            technique, needed to relieve allergic reaction
            symptoms suffered by patients.

Method: Data gathered and analyzed from office docu-
            mentation spanning a ten-year period. Data from
            both male and female subjects of various ages
            were used. The patients completed symptom
            survey questionnaires; 15 complaints represent-
            ing the most common signs/symptoms recorded
            in the sample group were used for the purpose of
            this analysis.

<u>The 15 most common complaints are:</u>

❑ Migraine Headache
❑ Fatigue
❑ Asthma
❑ Backache
❑ Indigestion
❑ Milk intolerance
❑ Excessive gas/bloating
❑ Constipation
❑ Diarrhea
❑ Insomnia
❑ Hot flashes
❑ Anxiety
❑ Depression
❑ Eczema
❑ PMS

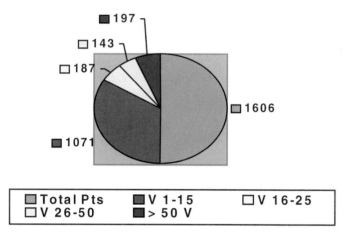

Figure 1

Migraine Headaches

66.7% of the patients complaining of
Migraine Headaches treated with **NAET**
had symptoms resolved within the first 15
visits.

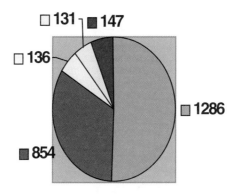

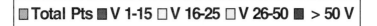

□ Total Pts ■ V 1-15 □ V 16-25 □ V 26-50 ■ > 50 V

Figure 2
Fatigue

66.4% of the patients complaining of
Fatigue treated with **NAET** had symptoms
resolved within the first 15 visits.

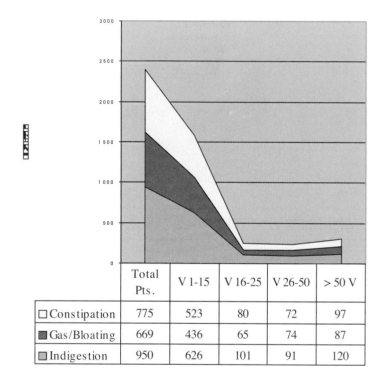

	Total Pts.	V 1-15	V 16-25	V 26-50	> 50 V
□ Constipation	775	523	80	72	97
■ Gas/Bloating	669	436	65	74	87
▨ Indigestion	950	626	101	91	120

Figure 3
Symptoms Resolved

* Less then 1.3% of patients failed to follow-up.

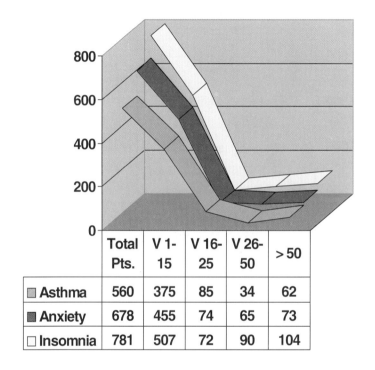

	Total Pts.	V 1-15	V 16-25	V 26-50	> 50
Asthma	560	375	85	34	62
Anxiety	678	455	74	65	73
Insomnia	781	507	72	90	104

Figure 4
Symptoms Resolved

* Less then 1.3% of patients failed to follow-up.

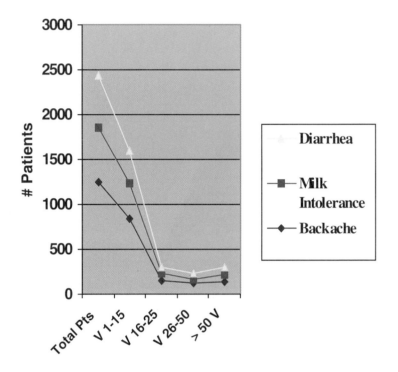

Figure 5
Symptoms Cleared

* Less then 1.3% of patients failed to follow-up

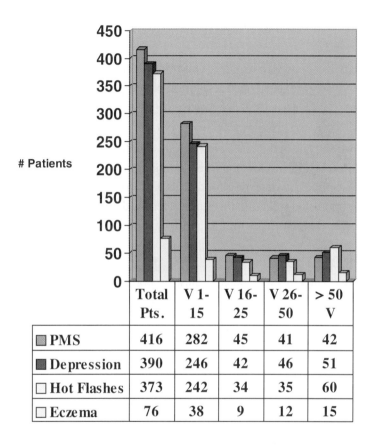

	Total Pts.	V 1-15	V 16-25	V 26-50	> 50 V
PMS	416	282	45	41	42
Depression	390	246	42	46	51
Hot Flashes	373	242	34	35	60
Eczema	76	38	9	12	15

Figure 6
Symptoms Resolved

* Less then 1.3% of patients failed to follow-up

The number of patient visits until symptoms resolved were then tracked and documented.

Results: Approximately two thirds of the sample group experienced resolution of symptoms within the first 15 visits. See figures 1-6.

In 1998, one of the kinesiology groups published a study on the effectiveness on Muscle Response Testing for allergies. MRT had 90.5% accuracy in detecting food allergies. I thought the readers will be interested to know this report. Here is the published study on Muscle Response Testing.

PILOT STUDY

Muscle testing to detect allergies is reported by the pilot study done by Water H. Schmitt, Jr. and Gerry Leisman, "Applied Neuroscience Laboratories," N.C., USA, and the College of Judea and Samaria, P.O.Box 3, Ariel, 44837, Israel entitled "Correlation of applied kinesiology muscle testing findings with serum immunoglobulin levels for food allergy," August 1998.

The pilot study attempted to determine whether subjective muscle testing employed by Applied Kinesiology practitioners, prospectively determine those individuals with specific hyperallergenic responses. Seventeen subjects were found positive on Applied Kinesiology (A.K.) muscle testing screening procedures indicating food hypersensitivity (allergy) reactions. Each subject showed muscle weakening (inhibition) reactions to oral provocative testing of one or two foods for a total of 21 positive food reactions. Tests for a hypersensitivity reaction of the serum were performed using both a radio-allergosorbent test (RAST) and immune complex test for IgE and IgG against all 21 of the foods that tested positive with A.K. muscle screening procedures. These serum tests confirmed 19 of the 21 food allergies (90.5%) suspected based on the applied kinesiology screening procedures. This pilot study offers a basis to examine further a means by which to predict the clinical utility of a given substance for a given patient, based on the patterns of neuromuscular response elicited from the patient, representing a conceptual expansion of the standard neurological examination process.

PMID: 10069623 [PubMed - indexed for MEDLINE]

It was more exciting when I was able to eat most food I wanted to eat, the food once made me extremely ill; wear regular clothes and feel normal. Within next few months of very dedicated, regular NAET treatments, I was able to get freedom from most food allergies, reactions, and most of all free from my nagging constant body aches and pains. I was free to eat, and free to wear different clothes (I lived on one pair of ragged clothes for five years, unable to wear anything else due to my body's severe allergic reaction to cotton, polyester and other materials). I was free to go to places, to travel, to fly in an airplane, visit places I'd always wanted to see. I had freedom to live without coughing and puffing, without crying in pain! I got a second chance for a normal life. Thank you God!

It was too good to be true to believe it initially. I thought I was dreaming and expected my pains and other illnesses to return any time. I do get occasional recurrences of some of my allergic reactions if I forget to check the item before I consume or use and if I happened to be still allergic to that item or never treated for it before. NAET clears allergies to all treated items. If something is not treated, if it is an allergen, you could still react to it when exposed. But I don't panic anymore since I can test using the testing techniques I have described in Chapter 6 and once detected, I can self-treat it and get free from the symptom instantly. Self-treatments are described in Chapter 8.

I need to cautioned you again that self-treatments should be tried only after one clears all the NAET Basic 15-20 allergens with a trained NAET practitioner.

MRT also detects the exact duration of avoidance. The body will diminish reaction to the allergen just by avoiding for the exact hours of avoidance after each NAET treatment. In most patients, the time of avoidance will be 24 to 25 hours. Some people with severe allergies may need more than 25 hours. I have also seen in a few people, the exact hours of avoidance was less than 24 hours. Needing less time may depend on a few factors: age (as a general rule, young ones may take less time), a good immune system, or living in a healthy environment, eating less polluted food, less allergic food, etc. The 25-hour avoidance will detoxify the entire system toward the treated allergen. When people do not follow the 25-hour (or more in some cases) avoidance after each treatment, we have noticed some minor side effects like recurrence of allergies, weight gain, etc. Because of this I recommend to all NAET patients to observe 25-hour avoidance period regardless of their immune system. If people follow proper NAET protocol, they need not go through specific, expensive, or time-consuming detoxification programs during or after completion of NAET treatments.

The brain is a very powerful and complicated organ. Information about the environment reaches the brain through various steps, mediated by neurotransmitters. A message begins its journey through the vast nervous system network, which consists of the autonomic nervous system, spinal cord, and brain. The journey begins as an impulse through the sympathetic and parasympathetic nervous systems, nociceptors, afferent and efferent nerve, spinal nerves, dorsal horn, five different ascending pathways, medulla, pons, cerebellum, midbrain, thalamus, hypothalamus, limbic system, corpus callosum, cerebral hemispheres, cerebrum, and association cortex. It returns through descending pathways to the target tissue and other associated tissues.

Through stimulation of a series of specific pressure points, NAET is able to send appropriate messages as impulses through ascending and descending pathways to the brain to reprogram the brain by removing the previously imprinted, inappropriate messages that resulted in allergies and allergy-based disorders, and re-imprinting with normal healthy messages.

The outcome of NAET is very satisfying for the patient as well as for the practitioner if it is done properly. It gives the patient the freedom to eat, drink, come in contact with items and environments that previously caused problems, and to lead a healthier life. It not only gives the practitioner the satisfaction of a job well done, but also of helping someone who might have suffered long periods of sickness with little relief.

Knowledge of Oriental medicine and acupuncture is an asset to understand NAET since various aspects of NAET treatment use Oriental medical knowledge. NAET also utilizes aspects of various other health disciplines, such as allopathy, chiropractic, naturopathy, nutritional, and traditional Western techniques.

NAET has not yet become standard medical practice. Over seven thousand medical practitioners from different fields of medicine have been trained in NAET. In addition to their success with patients, many of them have begun researches and clinical trials in their offices to prove the efficacy of NAET to the rest of the world.

CHAPTER 3

Categories of Allergens

Common allergens are generally classified into nine basic categories based primarily on the method in which they are contacted, rather than the symptoms they produce.

1. Inhalants

2. Ingestants

3. Contactants

4. Injectants

5. Infectants

6. Physical agents

7. Genetic factors

8. Molds and fungi

9. Emotional stressors

Inhalants

Inhalants are those allergens that are contacted through the nose, throat and bronchial tubes. Examples of inhalants are microscopic spores of certain grasses, flowers, pollens, mold, powders, smoke, cosmetics, perfumes; and chemical fumes such as paint, insecticides, fertilizers, flour from grains, cooking smells, etc.

Many people suffer from various types of nasal allergies with different intensities. Some of the common allergy-based respiratory problems are allergic rhinitis, bleeding from the nose, bronchitis, bronchial asthma, bronchospasms, cough, shortness of breath, dust allergy, frequent colds and influenzas, hay-fever, occupational asthma and pneumonia, viral and bacterial pneumonia, chemical pneumonia, post nasal drip, sinusitis, and certain respiratory tract infections.

Ingestants

Ingestants are allergens contacted in the normal course of eating a meal or enter the system in other ways through the mouth and find their way into the gastrointestinal tract. These include: foods, drinks, condiments, drugs, beverages, chewing gums, vitamin supplements, etc. We must not ignore the potential reactions to things that may be touched and inadvertently transmitted into the mouth by our hands.

The area of ingested allergens is one of the hardest to diagnose, because the allergic responses are often delayed from several minutes to several days, making direct association between cause and effect very difficult. This is not to say that an immediate response is not possible. Some people can react violently in seconds after they consume the allergens. In extreme cases, one has only to touch or come near the allergen to signal the central nervous system that it is about to be poisoned, resulting in symptoms that are peculiar to that particular patient. Usually, more violent reactions are observed in ingested allergens than in other forms.

Contactants

Contactants produce their effect by direct contact with the skin. They include the well-known poison oak, poison ivy, poison sumac, cats, dogs, and rabbits, but also cosmetics, soaps, detergents, fabric softeners, hair conditioner, shampoo, skin cream, rubbing alcohol, gloves, hair dyes, various types of plant oils, chemicals such as gasoline, dyes, acrylic nails, nail polish, fabrics (everyday attire, night clothes, bed linen, bath towels, bath tub toys, stuffed animals, books, newspaper, ink, formaldehyde, furniture, cabinets, etc.

Allergic reactions to contactants can be different in each person, and may include:

Asthma, constipation, cough, eczema, fainting spells, frequent urination, hives, insomnia, joint pains, mental confusion, mental irritability, migraine headaches, skin cancer, skin rashes, stomach aches, swelling of the body, various kinds of arthritis.

It is apparent that some allergens contacted by the skin can produce symptoms as devastating to the patient as anything ingested or inhaled.

Allergy to Fabrics

People can be allergic to the clothes they wear daily. We had seen patients who had allergy to cotton, nylon, and other synthetic fabrics. Woolen clothes may also cause allergies. We have seen people who cannot wear wool without breaking out in rashes. Some people who are sensitive to wool also react to creams with a lanolin base, since lanolin is derived from sheep's wool. Some people can be allergic to cotton socks, orlon socks, or woolen socks with symptoms of knee pain, etc. People can also be allergic to carpets and drapes that could cause knee pains and joint pains.

Persistent Yeast Infections in Females

We had a few female patients who were allergic to their panty hose and suffered from leg cramps, high blood pressure, swollen legs, psoriasis, and persistent yeast infections. Toilet paper and paper towels also cause problems, mimicking yeast infections in many people.

Allergy to Cosmetics

Many people are allergic to underarm deodorants and antiperspirants, causing skin rashes, irritation of the skin, dermatitis, boils, infections, lymph gland swelling and pain. The chemicals in the antiperspirants and deodorants are toxic and carcinogenic to some people. These products do their intended job to prevent sweating, by blocking the sweat glands. That could lead to inflammation of the sweat glands, and constant irritation and inflammation can lead to more chronic disorders like lymph blockage and breast cancer.

Many women are allergic to their synthetic bras and to feminine tampons. Reports from women-sufferers confirm that allergy to antiperspirant or usage of synthetic bras probably caused some of them to have fibrocystic breasts, breast lumps, breast cancers, and that tampons might have caused cervical cancer.

In the case of skin cancer, the causative factor may not only be overexposure to the sun, as many people think, but may be due to allergies to suntan lotion, skin cream, shaving cream, razor blades (stainless steel), clothing or other allergenic products. Consistent use of these products may well cause skin irritation or even skin cancer.

Allergy to Drugs

Sometimes cancer patients are allergic to the drugs they are taking to destroy cancer. If they are allergic to the chemotherapy drugs, or vitamins, minerals, or other supplements, these should be treated using NAET methods prior to using them. Thus, the side effects arising from allergies to the drugs or supplements can be eliminated and the drugs can work on the body to destroy the disease without any interference.

Heavy Metals

Heavy metal toxicity is on the rise. Most foods are sprayed with pesticides. Pesticides are loaded with heavy metals like mercury. Mercury is a neurotoxin that is the reason it is used in most pesticides to help immobilize the pests. Mercury is a neurotoxin in humans too. People can get exposed to mercury from dental fillings, childhood immunizations, fish and pesticides. Pressed wood, decorative woodwork, and some furniture are treated with pesticide derivatives to increase longevity.

Crude Oil

Many people are allergic to crude oils and their derivatives, which include plastic and synthetic rubber products. One cannot imagine the difficulty of living in this modern society, trying to be completely free from products made of crude oil. A person would literally be immobilized. The phones we use, the naugahyde chairs we sit on, the milk containers we use, the polyester fabrics we wear, most of the face and body creams we use, are all made from a common product—crude oil.

Sick Building Syndrome

Formaldehyde is found in fabrics, newspaper, ink, pressed wood, sheet rock, building materials, new carpet, name tags on the clothes, paints, etc. Many people have been diagnosed as suffering from "sick-building syndrome." People who work in the newspaper industry, and writers suffer from carpal tunnel syndrome, which is often an allergy to formaldehyde or plastic.

Other career-produced allergies have been diagnosed for cooks (spices, cooking oil smells), waiters (smell of the foods, plastic trays), grocery store employees or workers or simply grocers (various items like chemicals, to fresh food found in the store), clerks (paper products, inks, liquid paper, permanent markers), gardeners (pesticides, herbicides, plants, tools, leaf-blowers), computer programmers (computer radiation, plastics, electrical cords, mouse, keyboard, monitor), teachers (white board, pens, markers, paper, glue), bakers (flour, eggs, baking powder, artificial colors, flavorings, food chemicals), surgeons (latex gloves, gowns, masks, surgical instruments, antiseptics), lawyers (paper, pens, markers, computers, books, leather chair, wood-office furniture, cell phones), etc. Virtually no trade or skill is exempt from being exposed to allergens.

Injectants

Allergens are injected into the skin, muscles, joints and blood vessels in the form of various serums, antitoxins, vaccines and drugs. As in any other allergic reaction, the injection of a sensitive drug into the system runs the risk of producing dangerous allergic reactions. To the sensitive person, the drug actively becomes a poison, with the same effect as an injection of arsenic. No medical professional would intentionally give an injection of a potentially dangerous drug to a person. However, some drugs seem to become more allergenic for certain people over time, without the person being aware of the potential future risk. The reaction to the drug penicillin is an example. The reactions vary, from hives to diarrhea to anaphylactic shock and death.

Insect bites and stings fall in this category. The toxic secretions of these insects are fatal to many sensitive people. Snake bite and bee sting fatalities are very common in tropical countries.

Infectants

Infectants are allergens that produce their effect by causing an adverse reaction to an infectious agent, such as bacteria. For example, when tuberculin test is introduced as part of a diagnostic test to determine a patient's sensitivity and/or reaction to that particular agent, an allergic reaction may result. Likewise, this may occur during skin patch testing, or from scratch tests done in the normal course of allergy testing in traditional Western medical procedure.

Various vaccinations and immunizations may also produce such allergic reactions. Some sensitive children, after they receive their usual immunizations, get very sick physically and emotionally.

Physical Agents and Physical Activities

Heat, cold, sunlight, dampness, dryness, humidity, drafts, fog, smog or mechanical irritants may also cause allergic reactions and are known as physical allergens. When the patient suffers from more than one allergy, physical agents can deeply affect the patient. If the patient has already eaten some allergic foods, then walks in cold air or drafts, he/she might develop upper respiratory problems, sore throat, asthma or joint pains, etc., depending on his tendency toward health-related problems. Some people are very sensitive to cold or heat, whether they have eaten any allergic food or not. Such cases are common.

Many patients with arthritis, asthma, migraine, PMS, as well as mental patients, have exaggerated symptoms on cold, cloudy or rainy days. These types of patients could suffer from severe allergy to electrolytes, cold, or a combination of both.

Some patients violently react to heat or cold, experiencing, body aches or joint pains during a cloudy day, and icy cold hands and feet even if they are clad in multiple warm socks. These patients have hypo-functioning immune systems. When they finish the NAET treatment program, they do not continue to feel cold or get sick from heat or cold.

Exercise is very important for the body to maintain proper circulation of blood and nutrients to the vital organs and to each and every cell of the body. Proper blood circulation is also important to eliminate toxins from the body. Healthy adrenal glands hold the key to better health by maintaining a healthy immune system. People with good immune system manifest less allergies.

People could be allergic to exercise. Exercise-induced asthma, migraines, anaphylaxis and death are seen more frequently since people are getting more involved with fitness programs around the country. Endorphins and enkephalins are produced in large amounts during exercise. These are the brain enzymes that produce a sense of well-being. It is possible for you to be allergic to your own endorphin and other hormones. People who get anaphylaxis during exercise may be allergic to their own endorphins. They should first get treated with NAET for endorphins and other specific hormones before they begin a vigorous exercise program.

Another option to vigorous exercise is Yoga. Yoga exercises are gentle, and can be practiced by anybody, weak or strong, young or old. These are specific exercises practiced regularly to strengthen weak vital organs. There are precise Yoga exercises to strengthen the adrenal glands and to stimulate the immune system. Since these exercises can stimulate the adrenals and maintain a good immune system, Yoga exercises will be very helpful in reducing allergies and allergy-related illnesses. It is an excellent program to help with any imbalances of the brain including brain allergies, brain fog, chemical sensitivities affecting brain, ADD, ADHD, Autism, learning disabilities, dyslexia, bipolar disorders, schizophrenia, manic disorders and depression. Very weak patients should begin with one or two Yoga exercises until they are strong enough to add more into their schedule. Exercise is a good way to expel toxins from specific organs, to reduce stress and to bring overall calmness. Yoga should not be practiced without proper knowledge or guidance. People with reactions to aerobics or other type of exercises should look into learning Yoga. It is taught in schools and universities. There are many Yoga centers around the country. Please find one near you and learn the exercises properly from a teacher.

Genetic Causes

Discovery of possible tendencies toward allergies carried over from parents and grandparents opens a large door to achieving optimum health. Most people inherit their allergic tendency from their parents or grandparents. Allergies can skip generations and be manifested very differently in children.

Many people with various allergic manifestations respond well to being treated for the various disease agents that have been transmitted from parents.

The number of people suffering from chronic fatigue syndrome and fibromyalgia is on the rise. People suffering from multiple chemical sensitivities are also increasing. We have seen genetic factors play a huge role in these types of ailments. Ancestors may have suffered from some infectious disorders and the toxins produced from the infection have caused genetic alteration in their genes. The altered genes were replicated and duplicated in future generations. Thus, the allergic tendency was handed down and the manifestation depended on the general condition of the offspring.

Parents with rheumatic fever may transmit disease possibilities to their offspring but in the children the rheumatic fever agent may not be manifested in its original form.

Molds and Fungi

Molds and fungi are in a category by themselves because of the numerous ways they are contacted as allergens in everyday experience. They can be ingested, inhaled, touched or even injected, as in the case of penicillin. They come in the form of airborne spores, making up a large part of the dust we breathe or pick up in our vacuum cleaners; fluids such as our drinking water; as dark fungal growth in the corners of damp rooms; as athlete's foot; and in particularly vaginal "yeast infections." They grow on trees and in the damp soil. They are a source of food, as in truffles and mushrooms; of diseases such as ringworm and the aforementioned yeast infections, and of healing, as in the tremendous benefits mankind has derived from the drug Penicillin.

Reactions to these substances are as varied as to other kinds of allergies. This is because they are a part of one of the largest known classifications of biological entities. Because of the number of ways they can be introduced into the human body, the reactions are multiplied considerably. Fungi are parasites that grow on living as well as decaying organic matter. That means that some forms are found growing in the human anatomy. The problem of athlete's foot is a prime example.

Athlete's foot is a human parasite fungus that grows anywhere in the area of body where it is moist for a long time and not exposed to sunlight or air. It is particularly difficult to eliminate, and treatment generally consists of a topical preparation, multiple daily cleansing of the area, a medicinal powder, and wearing light cotton socks or other clothing, to avoid further infection from dyes used in colored wearing apparel.

It is contracted by contact with the fungus and is often passed from person to person anywhere there is the potential for contact (i.e. gymnasium, showers, locker rooms and other areas where people share facilities and walk barefoot), thus the name athlete's foot. If it is a real athlete's foot, it will clear with the NAET treatment. Certain allergies, like allergies to socks made of cotton, orlon, or nylon, etc., can mimic athlete's foot. In such cases, athlete's foot may not clear by using medications, and must be treated by NAET for allergy to such fabrics.

Allergies to cotton, orlon, nylon, or paper could result in the explosions of infections including ascomycetes fungi (yeast) that women find so troublesome. Feminine tampons, toilet papers, douches, and deodorants can also cause yeast infections.

Emotional Stressors

The origin of physical or physiological symptoms can often be traced back to some unresolved emotional trauma, or to some misunderstood stress in one or more of the energy pathways. Each cell in the body (meridians) has the capability to respond physically, physiologically and psychologically to our daily activities. When the vital energy flows evenly and uninterrupted through the energy pathways (acupuncture meridians), the body functions normally. When there is a disruption in the energy flow through the meridians (an increase or decrease), energy blockages can occur, causing various symptoms in those particular meridians.

Using the existing knowledge about the human body from Eastern and Western perspectives, one can access the information about the stressed tissue, organ or even a cell in the body. An NAET practitioner will use these categories of allergens to try to detect the cause of health problems, as well as which specific tissue is being affected by the invader, whether it may be an inhalant, ingestant, contactant, infectant (pathogen), physical agent, genetic agent, or other stressor.

CHAPTER 4

Detecting Allergies

Allergic conditions occur much more frequently than most people realize. Every year there are more and more recognized cases of allergies in the United States. Statistics show that at least 50 percent of the population suffers from some form of allergy. Many people are interested in understanding the differences and/or the similarities of the methods of diagnosis, the effectiveness and length of treatment between traditional Western medicine and Oriental medicine. Since the purpose of this book is to provide information about the new treatment method of NAET, more attention will be given to Oriental medicine.

With NAET, it is extremely important for the patient to cooperate with the physician in order to obtain the best results. It is my hope that this chapter will help bring about a clearer understanding between allergists and their patients because, in order to obtain the most satisfactory results, both parties must work together as a team.

The first step in diagnosing an allergy is to take a thorough patient history, including chief complaint, present history, past medical history, family history, social history, history of activities, hobbies and nutrition. It will be beneficial to obtain a thorough record of any allergic symptoms in the patient's family, tracing back two or three generations if possible. The patient will be asked whether either parent suffers from asthma or hay fever, ever suffered from hives, reacted to a serum injection (such as tetanus antitoxin, DPT), or experienced any type of skin trouble. Additionally, the allergist will ask whether the patient's parents were unable to eat certain foods or professed to "hate" certain foods because of how the particular food made them feel; complained of sinusitis, runny nose, frequent colds or flu; had dyspepsia, indigestion, mental illness, heart disorders, skin disorders, or any other conditions where an allergy may have been a contributing factor, whether or not recognized as such at the time.

The same questions are asked about the patient's other relatives: grandparents, aunts, uncles, brothers, sisters and cousins. An allergic tendency is not always inherited directly from the parents. It may skip generations, and manifest in nieces or nephews rather than in direct descendants.

The careful allergist will also determine whether such diseases as tuberculosis, cancer, diabetes, rheumatic or glandular disorders exist or have ever occurred in the patient's family history. All of these facts help give the allergist a more complete picture of the hereditary characteristics of the patient. *Allergic tendency* is inherited. It may be manifested differently in different people. Unlike the tendency, an actual allergic condition, such as asthma, is not always inherited. Parents may have had cancer or rheumatism, but the child can manifest that allergic inheritance as asthma.

When the family history is complete, the allergist will need to look into the history of the patient's allergic attacks. Some typical preliminary questions include: When did your first attack occur? Did your allergy first occur when you were an infant or a child, or did you first notice the symptoms after you were fully grown? Did it occur after going through a certain procedure? For example, did it occur for the first time after a dental procedure like a root canal? One of my patients reported that her asthma occurred for the first time four hours after root canal work. She was allergic to *Gutta*

Percha Tissue that was used in the procedure.

Once a careful history is taken, the allergist often discovers that the patient's first symptoms occurred in early childhood. He or she may have suffered from infantile eczema, but never associated it with asthma which may not have appeared until middle age.

Next, the doctor will want to know the circumstances surrounding and immediately preceding the first symptoms. Typical questions will include: Did you change your diet or go on a special diet? Did you eat something that you hadn't eaten perhaps for two or three months? Do you eat one type of food repeatedly, every day? Did the symptoms follow a childhood illness (whooping cough, measles, chicken pox, diphtheria) or any immunization for such an illness? Did they follow some other illness, such as influenza, pneumonia, viral infection, or a major operation? Did the symptoms first appear at adolescence or after you had a baby? Were they first noticed after you acquired a cat, a dog, or even a bird? Did they appear after an automobile accident or any major physical or mental trauma? Did they appear after a lengthy exposure to the sun, a day at the beach or 18 holes of golf? Did they appear after receiving a gift for your birthday? Or after starting to use a new pair of socks, pants, shirt, after-shave, wrist watch, leather belt, leather shoes, a chair, furniture, certain shampoo, cosmetics? Did your symptoms begin after a new arrival in the house (a baby, a guest, a pet, etc.)?

Any one of these factors can be responsible for triggering a severe allergic manifestation or precipitate the first noticeable symptoms of an allergic condition. Therefore, it is very important to obtain full and accurate answers when taking a patient's medical history.

Other important questions relate to the frequency and occurrence of the attacks. Although foods may be a factor, if the symptoms occur only at specific times of the year, the trouble is most likely due to pollens. Often a patient is sensitive to certain foods but has a natural tolerance that prevents sickness until the pollen sensitivity adds sufficient allergens to throw the body into an imbalance. If symptoms occur only on specific days of the week, they are probably due to something contacted or eaten on that particular day.

The causes of allergic attacks in different patients can, at first, appear to be random. Regular weekly attacks of sneezing and nasal allergy were the effects in one patient after he read the Sunday newspaper. The ink caused a severe allergic reaction. Another patient reacted similarly to the comic section of the newspaper. A man always had a gastrointestinal allergic attack on Sunday morning. The cause was traced to eating a traditional pizza every Saturday night with his family. He was allergic to the tomato sauce on the pizza. Still another patient had an allergic attack of sneezing and runny nose on Saturdays. I traced the allergy to the chemical compounds in a lotion she used to set her hair on Friday afternoons.

The time of day when the attacks occur is also of importance in determining the cause of an allergic manifestation. If it always occurs at night, it is quite likely that there is something in the bedroom that is aggravating the condition. It may be that the patient is sensitive to feathers in the pillow or comforter, wood cabinets, marble floors, carpets, side tables, end tables, bed sheets, pillows, pillow cases, detergents used in washing clothes, indoor plants, or shrubs, trees or grasses outside the patient's window.

Many patients react violently to house dust, different types of furniture, polishes, house plants, tap water and purified water. Most city water suppliers change the water chemicals only once or twice a year. Although this is done with good intentions, people with chemical allergies may get sicker if they ingest the same chemicals over and over for months or years.

Contrary to traditional Western thinking, developing immunity can be the exception rather than the rule.

Occasionally, switching foods, chemicals or other substances gives a change of allergens to an allergic patient and a chance for him/her to recover from reactions. In this way, some allergies can be avoided.

Drinking water comes from different sources. The major sources are ground water and surface water. The ground water supply includes underground aquifers, wells and springs. Most aquifers get their water supply from surface water, which includes lakes, ponds and rivers. Dumping contaminants into the water or onto the soil contaminates both sources. The soil contaminants are carried either throughout the soil to the underground source (such as wells and springs), or through the runoff of the contaminated soil into lakes and rivers.

Contamination may also be caused by natural degradation of vegetation, animal matter or pollutants in the air and in rain. Surface water can also be tainted via contaminated lakes, rivers and ponds through direct dumping of pollutants from accidental spills, pesticides, septic tank cesspools, landfills, dump or refuse spills, gasoline or diesel spills, industrial disposals, bacteria, virus and parasites (roundworms, hookworms and tapeworms).

The amount and strength of the pollutants and disinfectants in the water vary. In any given region, after the first heavy rain, we usually see an epidemic of influenza in that area.

The doctor should ask the patient to make a daily log of all the foods he/she is eating. The ingredients in the food should be checked for possible allergens. Certain common allergens like corn products, MSG (monosodium glutamate or Accent), citric acid, etc., are used in many food preparations.

Allergy to corn is one of today's most common allergies, especially in asthmatic and arthritic patients. Unfortunately, cornstarch is found in almost every processed food and some toiletries and drugs as well. Chinese food, baking soda, baking powder and toothpaste contain large amounts of cornstarch. It is the binding product in almost all vitamins and pills, including aspirin and Tylenol. Corn syrup is the natural sweetener in many of the products we ingest, including soft drinks. Corn silk is found in cosmetics and corn oil is used as a vegetable oil. Cotton crotches of female underpants are treated with baking soda and baking powder for better hygiene. But an allergy to corn from baking soda is found to be one of the common sources of never-ending yeast-like infections in women. Many women became free of yeast-like infections after treating for cornstarch with NAET.

People react severely to various gums used in many preparations: Acacia gum, xanthine gum, karaya gum, etc. Numerous gums are used in candy bars, yogurt, cream cheese, soft drinks, soy sauce, barbecue sauce, fast food products, macaroni and cheese, etc.

Carob, a staple in many health food products, is another item that causes many common diseases among allergic people. Many health—conscious people are turning to natural food products in which carob is used as a chocolate and cocoa substitute. It is also used as a natural coloring or stiffening agent in soft drinks, cheeses, sauces, etc. We discovered that some of the causes of "holiday flu" are allergies to carob, chocolate and turkey.

After completing the patient's history, allergists should examine the patient for the usual vital signs. A physical examination is performed to check for any abnormal growth or condition. If the patient has an area of pain or discomfort in the body, it should be inspected. It is important to identify the type of pain, the location of the pain, and its relation to an acupuncture point. Excluding traumas, most pain in the body usually occurs around some important acupuncture point.

Nambudripad's Testing Techniques (NTT)

NAET uses many standard allopathic and kinesiological testing procedures to detect allergies. Some of the common ones are mentioned below.

1. History

A complete history of the patient is taken. A symptom survey form is given to the patient to record the level and type of discomfort he/she is suffering.

2. Physical Examination

Observation of the mental status, face, skin, eyes, color, posture, movements, gait, tongue, scars, wounds, marks, body secretions, etc.

3. Vital Signs

Evaluation of blood pressure, pulse, skin temperature and palpable pains in the course of meridians, etc.

4. NAETER (Electro-Dermal Test-EDT) or SRT

Skin Resistance Test for the presence or absence of a suspected allergen is done through a computerized electrodermal testing device; differences in the meter reading are observed (the greater the difference, the stronger the allergy).

5. MRT

Muscle Response Testing is conducted to compare the strength of a predetermined muscle in the presence and absence of a suspected allergen. If the particular muscle (test muscle) weakens in the presence of an item, it signifies that the item is an allergen. If the muscle remains strong, the substance is not an allergen. More explanation on MRT will be given in Chapter 6.

6. Dynamometer Testing

A hand-held dynamometer is used to measure finger strength (0-100 scale) in the presence and absence of a suspected allergen. The dynamometer is held with thumb and index finger and squeezed to make the reading needle swing between 0-100 scale. An initial baseline reading is observed first, then the allergen is held and another reading taken. The finger strength is compared in the presence of the allergen. If the second reading is more than the initial reading, there is no allergy. If the second reading is less than the initial reading, then there is an allergy.

7. EMF Test (Electro Magnetic Field Test)

The electromagnetic component of the human energy field can be detected with simple muscle response testing. The pool of electromagnetic energy around an object or a person allows the energy exchange. The human field absorbs the energy from the nearby object and processes it through the network of nerve energy pathways. If the foreign energy field shares suitable charges with the human energy field, the human field absorbs the foreign energy for its advantage and becomes stronger. If the foreign energy field carries unsuitable charges, the human energy field causes repulsion of the foreign energy field. These types of reactions of the human field can be determined by testing an indicator muscle (specific muscle) before and after coming in contact with an allergen. The electromagnetic field of the human, or the human vibrations, can also be measured by using the sophisticated electronic equipment developed by Dr. Valerie Hunt of Malibu, California, a retired UCLA physics professor, has proven her theory of the Science of Human Vibrations through 25 years of extensive research and clinical studies. Her book, "Infinite Mind," explains it all.

8. Pulse Test

Pulse testing is another simple way of determining food allergy. This test was developed by Arthur Coca, M.D. in the

1950's. Research has shown that if you are allergic to something and you eat it, your pulse rate speeds up.

Step 1: Establish your base-line pulse by counting radial pulse at the wrist for a full minute.

Step 2: Put a small portion of the suspected allergen in the mouth, preferably under the tongue. Taste the substance for two minutes. Do not swallow any portion of it. The taste will send the signal to the brain, which will send a signal through the sympathetic nervous system to the rest of the body.

Step 3: Retake the pulse with the allergen still in the mouth. An increase or decrease in pulse rate of 10% or more is considered an allergic reaction. The greater the degree of allergy, the greater the difference in the pulse rate.

This test is useful to test food allergies. If you are allergic to very many foods, and if you consume a few allergens at the same time, it will be hard to detect the exact allergen causing the reaction just by this test.

9. NAET Rotation Diet

After clearing the allergy to the basic NAET allergens, the foods from the allergy-free list is consumed in a pre-selected order. Then use the question response test (ask questions while doing MRT and muscle weakness will be interpreted as "yes" answer, and a muscle strength will be interpreted as "no" answer. Every meal is selected from a non-allergic list according to the priority. This prevents overload of the particular food in the body and reduces unwanted allergic reactions and allergy-based disorders.

10. Hold, Sit and Test

This is a simple procedure to test allergies. Place a small portion of the suspected allergen in a baby food jar or thin-glass jar, preferably with a lid, then the person will hold it in her/his palm, touching the jar with the fingertips of the same hand for 15 to 30 minutes. If the person is allergic to the item in the jar, he/she will begin to feel uneasy when holding the allergen in the palm, giving rise to various unpleasant symptoms. This testing procedure is described in detail in Chapter 8. When we treat patients who have a history of anaphylaxis to a particular item, we use this method after completing the required NAET treatments and before the patient begins to use the item again.

If the patient was treated for a severe peanut allergy, (or milk, egg, wheat, fish, mushroom, etc.) after going through the required NAET treatments to neutralize the peanut, the patient is allowed to sit and hold the peanuts in a glass jar every day for 30 minutes for three days to a week. If the patient does not show any symptoms of previous allergy, he/she will be allowed to hold a peanut in the hand without a bottle for three to five days, 30 minutes daily. If that does not produce any allergic reaction, then the patient will be allowed to put a small piece of nut in the mouth and hold it there for five to ten minutes every day for a few days. If that also does not produce any reaction, the patient will be allowed to eat a small piece of the nut and observe the reaction. Usually, by this time, the patient will be able to use the allergen confidently without fear. Check with your practitioner for more details.

11. Positive Inputs

In order to achieve a particular goal in your life, you must make sure that your computer (in this case, your brain) is programmed correctly. You can open up your database of your brain computer and inspect it carefully for any self-damaging type of information that may exist in any part of the program. Using MRT, you can open up your computer and inspect it for sabotaged programs. Sometimes, the whole brain may not keep the sabotaging memory, but just an organ, a limb, a specific tissue of the brain, a major artery, nerve, a part of the body, may hold on to the damaging memory that happened years ago and can cause a problem forever. One can use MRT to detect the damaged tissue or organ. Once inspected, the incorrect program can be fixed through NAET. It may be time-consuming, but it is worth doing if you want to live a healthier life. Check with your NAET doctor.

Commonly Used Standard Laboratory Tests

12. ALCAT Test

One of today's most reliable and effective blood tests to detect allergies and sensitivities to food, chemicals, and food additives is the ALCAT test. This system is designed to measure blood cell reactions to foods, chemicals, drugs, molds, pesticides, bacteria, etc.

13. Scratch Test

Western medical allergists generally depend on skin testing (scratch test, patch test, etc.), in which a very small amount of a suspected allergic substance is introduced into the person's skin through a scratch or an injection. The site of injection is observed for any reaction. If there is any reaction at the area of injection, the person is considered to be allergic to that substance. Each item has to be tested individually.

14. Intradermal Test

A small portion of the extract of the allergen is injected intradermally, between the superficial layers of skin. Many people who show no reaction to the dermal or scratch type of testing show positive results when the same allergens are applied intradermally.

15. Radioallergosorbant Test (RAST)

The RAST measures IgE antibodies in serum and identifies specific allergens causing allergic reactions.

16. ELISA

Another blood serum test for allergies is called the "ELISA" (enzyme-linked immuno-zorbent assay) test. In this test, blood serum is tested for various immunoglobulin and their concentrations.

17. Cytotoxic Testing

Cytotoxic testing is a form of blood test. In this method, an extract of the allergic substance is mixed with a sample of the person's blood. It is then observed under the microscope for changes in white cells.

18. Elimination Diet

The elimination diet, which was developed by Dr. Albert H. Rowe of Oakland, California, consists of a very limited diet that must be followed for a period long enough to determine whether or not any of the foods included in it are responsible for the allergic symptoms. The importance of adhering strictly to the diet during the diagnostic period is very crucial. When the patient has been free of symptoms for a specific period, other foods are added, one at a time, until a normal diet is attained and the offending foods are discovered.

19. Rotation Diet

Another way to test for food allergy is through a "rotation diet," in which a different group of foods are consumed every day for a week. This will work for people with mild to moderate amount of allergies. This may not work well with people with severe allergies.

CHAPTER 5

The Brain-Body Connection

The human body is made up of bones, flesh, nerves and blood vessels, which can only function in the presence of vital energy. Like electricity, vital energy is not visible to the human eye.

No one knows how or why the vital energy gets into the body or how, when or where it goes when it leaves. It is true, however, that without it, none of the body functions can take place. When the human body is alive, vital energy flows freely through the energy pathways. Uninterrupted circulation of the vital energy flowing through the energy pathways keeps the person alive. This circulation of energy makes all the body functions possible. The circulation of the vital energy circulation makes the blood travel through the blood vessels, helping to distribute appropriate nutrients to various parts of the body for its growth, development, functions, and for repair of wear and tear.

NAET has its origin in Oriental medicine. But if one explores all the Oriental medical books, acupuncture textbooks, one may not find the NAET interpretation or evaluation about health problems that I write in my books anywhere else, because NAET is my sole development after observing my own reactions, my family's and patients' over the past two decades. Information about acupuncture meridians are kept to a minimum, enough to educate the reader about some of their traditional functions and possible dysfunctions in the presence of energy disturbances. Some of this information is also available in acupuncture textbooks that one may find in libraries. One needs to have some understanding about NAET evaluation of allergies and allergy-related disorders using Oriental medical knowledge to understand NAET. If anyone wishes to learn more about acupuncture meridians and mind-body connections in detail, please read Chapter 10 in my book, "Say Good-bye to Illness."

NAET utilizes a variety of standard medical procedures to diagnose allergies and then to treat allergies and allergy-related health conditions. These include: standard medical diagnostic procedures and standard allergy testing procedures (read Chapter 4) and an electro-dermal computerized allergy testing machine to detect allergies. After detecting allergies, NAET uses standard, chiropractic and acupuncture/acupressure treatments to eliminate allergies. Various studies have proven that NAET is capable of erasing the previously encoded incorrect message about an allergen and replacing it with a harmless or useful message by reprogamming the brain. This is accomplished by bringing the body into a state of "homeostasis" using other NAET energy balancing techniques.

Chiropractic theory postulates that a pinch or obstruction in one or more of the spinal nerve roots may cause nerve energy disturbance in the body causing poor nerve energy supply to target organs. When the particular nerves system fail to supply adequate amounts of energy to the organs and tissues, normal functions and appropriate enzymatic functions do not take place. The affected organs and tissues then begin to manifest impaired functions in digestion, absorption, assimilation and elimination. An allergy also causes impaired functions of the organs and tissues in one's body. Chiropractically speaking, an allergy can be seen as a result of a pinched nerve. Impaired functions of the organs and tissues will improve when the pinching of the spinal nerves is removed and energy circulation is restored.

Oriental medical theory explains the same thing from a different perspective. In Oriental medicine, the Yin-Yang state represents the perfect balance of energies (the state of homeostasis) in one's body. Any interference in the energy flow or an energy disturbance can cause an imbalance in the Yin-Yang state and an imbalance in "Homeostasis." Any substance that is capable of creating an energy disturbance in one's body is called an allergen. The result of this energy disturbance is called an allergy.

According to the NAET theory, when a substance is brought into the electro-magnetic field of a person, an attraction or repulsion takes place between the energy of the person and the substance.

Attraction

If two energies are attracted to each other, both energies are good to each other. The living person can benefit from the association of the other substance. The energy of the substance will combine with the person and enhance the functional ability of the person many fold. For example: After taking an antibiotic, the bacterial infection is diminished in a few hours. Here the energy of the antibiotic joined forces with the energy of the body and helped to eliminate the bacteria. Another example is taking vitamin supplements and the gaining of energy and vitality.

Repulsion

If two energies are repelling from each other, they are not good for each other. The living person can experience the repulsion of his/her energy from the other one as some discomfort in the body. The energy of the person will cause energy blockages in his/her energy meridians in the pretext to prevent the invasion of the adverse energy into the person's energy field. For example: After taking an antibiotic, not only the bacterial infection didn't get better and the person breaks out in a rash all over the body causing fever, nausea, excessive perspiration, lightheadedness, etc. Another example is taking vitamin supplements one night and waking up with multiple joint pains and general body-ache next morning. If repulsion takes place between two energies, then the substance that is capable of producing the repulsion in a living person is called an allergen. When the allergen produces a repulsion of energy in the electro-magnetic field, certain energy disturbance takes place in the body. The energy disturbance caused from the repulsion of the substance is capable of producing various unpleasant or adverse reactions in the body. These reactions are called "allergic reactions."

Immunoglobulins

In certain instances, the body also produces many defensive forces like "Histamine, immunoglobulins, etc." to help the body to overcome the unpleasant reactions from the interaction with the allergen. Most common immunoglobulin produced during these reactions is called IgE (immunoglobulinE). These reactions are called IgE-mediated reactions. During certain reactions, specific immunoglobulins are not produced. These are called non-IgE mediated reactions. Different types of immunoglobulins are produced during allergic reactions.

An allergy means an altered reactivity. This altered reactivity can happen between two people; between one person and a non-living substance; between one person and many non-living substances; between one person and a living person plus one or more non-living substances, etc.

These reactions and after-effects can be measured using various standard medical diagnostic tests. Energy medicine has also developed various devices to measure the reactions. Oriental medicine has used "I Ching" almost for the same purpose since 3,322

BC. Another simple way to test one's body is through simple, kinesiological muscle response testing (MRT) procedures. It is an easy procedure to evaluate the daily progress of the patient.

Study of the acupuncture meridians is necessary to understand muscle response testing and how it works. If one learns to identify the abnormal symptoms connected with the acupuncture meridians, detection of allergens will be easier. The pathological functions of the twelve major acupuncture meridians (energy disturbance) are given below.

THE LUNG MERIDIAN (LU)

Energy disturbance in the lung meridian affecting physical and physiological levels can give rise to the following symptoms:

Afternoon fever, asthma between 3-5 a.m., atopic dermatitis, bronchitis, bronchiectasis, burning in the eyes, burning in the nostrils, cardiac asthma, chest congestion, cough, coughing up blood, cradle cap, dry mouth, dry throat, dry skin, emaciated look, emphysema, profuse perspiration, morning fatigue, fever with chills, frequent flu-like symptoms, headache between eyes, general body ache with burning sensation, generalized hives, hair loss, hair thinning, hay-fever, infantile eczema, infection in the respiratory tract, itching of the nostrils, itching of the body, itching of the scalp, lack of perspiration, lack of desire to talk, laryngitis, low voice, night sweats, mucus in the throat, nasal congestion, nose bleed, pain in the chest and intercostal muscles, between third and fourth thoracic vertebrae, in the first interphalangeal joint, in the upper first and second cuspids (tooth), in the thumb, in the upper back, in the eyes, and in the upper arms; pleurisy, pharyngitis, pneumonia, poor growth of nails and hair, postnasal drip, red cheeks, red eyes, restlessness between 3 to 5 a.m., runny nose with clear discharge, thin or thick white discharge in case of viral infection, thick yellow discharge in case of bacterial infection, tonsillitis, scaly and rough skin, skin rashes, skin tags, moles, sinus infections, sinus headaches, sneezing, sore throat, stuffy nose, swollen throat, swollen cervical glands, tenosynovitis, throat irritation, warts, and inability to sleep after 3 am.

Energy disturbance in the lung meridian affecting the cellular level can cause the following:

Cellular level blockage of lung meridian often expresses grief or sadness. When one fails to cry, when one feels deep sorrow, sadness will settle in the lungs and eventually cause various lung disorders. Other symptoms of cellular level imbalance: Apologizing, comparing self with others, contempt, dejection, depression, despair, false pride, hopelessness, intolerance, likes to humiliate others, loneliness, low self-esteem, meanness, melancholy, over sympathy, over demanding, prejudice, seeking others' approval in doing things, self pity, highly sensitive emotionally, and weeping frequently without much reason.

Essential nutrients to strengthen the lung meridian:

Clear water, proteins, vitamin C, bioflavonoid, cinnamon, onions, garlic, B-vitamins (especially B_2), citrus fruits, green peppers, black peppers and rice.

THE LARGE INTESTINE MERIDIAN (LI)

Energy disturbance in the large intestine meridian affecting physical and physiological levels can give rise to the following symptoms:

Abdominal pain, acne on the face especially sides of the mouth and nose, asthma after 5 a.m., arthritis of the shoulder joint, arthritis of the knee joint, arthritis of the index finger, arthritis of the wrist joint, arthritis of the lateral part of the elbow and hip, bad breath, blisters in the lower gum, bursitis, dermatitis, dry mouth and thirst, eczema, fatigue, feeling better after a bowel movement, or feeling tired after a bowel movement, flatulence, inflammation of lower gum, intestinal colic, itching of the body, loose stools or constipation, lower backache, headaches, muscle spasms and pain of lateral thigh and knee, motor impairment of the fingers, pain in the knee, pain in the shoulder and shoulder blade, back of the neck, pain and swelling of the index finger, pain in the lateral aspect of the leg below the knee joint, pain in the heel, sciatic pain, swollen cervical glands, skin rashes, skin tags, sinusitis, tenosynovitis, tennis elbow, toothache, warts on the skin.

Energy disturbance in the large intestine meridian affecting the cellular level can cause the following:

Guilt, constipation of the mind, bad dreams, dwelling on past memory, crying spells, defensiveness, inability to recall dreams, nightmares, nostalgia, rolling restlessly in sleep, sadness, seeking sympathy, talking in the sleep and weeping.

Essential nutrients to strengthen the large intestine meridian:

Vitamins A, D, E, C, B, especially B_1, wheat, wheat bran, oat bran, yogurt, and roughage.

THE STOMACH MERIDIAN (ST)

Energy disturbance in the stomach meridian affecting physical and physiological levels can give rise to the following symptoms:

Abdominal distention, acid reflux disorders, acne on the face and neck, ADD, ADHD, anorexia, Autism, bad breath, black and blue marks on the leg below the knee, bipolar disorders, blemishes, bulimia, chest muscle pain, coated tongue, coldness in the lower limbs, cold sores in the mouth, delirium, depression, dry nostrils, dyslexia, facial paralysis, fever blisters, fibromyalgia, flushed face, frontal headache, heat boils (painful, reddish, acne) in the upper front of the body, herpes, hiatal hernia, high fever, learning disability, insomnia due to nervousness, itching on the skin below the knee, migraine headaches, manic depressive disorders, nasal polyps, nausea, nosebleed, pain on the upper jaws, pain in the mid-back, pain in the eye, persistent hunger, red rashes, seizures, sensitivity to cold, sore throat, sore tongue, sores on the gums, stomach ache, sweating, swelling on the neck, temporomandibular joint problem, unable to relax the mind or stop thinking, upper gum diseases and vomiting.

Energy disturbance in the stomach meridian affecting the cellular level can cause the following:

Disgust, bitterness, aggressive behaviors, attention deficit disorders, butterfly sensation in the stomach, constant thinking, depression, deprivation, despair, disappointment, egotism, emptiness, greed, hyperactivity, manic disorder, mental fog, mental confusion, nervousness, nostalgia, obsession, paranoia, poor concentration, poor memory, restlessness and schizophrenia.

Essential nutrients to strengthen the stomach meridian:

B complex especially B_{12}, B_6, B_3 and folic acid.

THE SPLEEN MERIDIAN (SP)

Energy disturbance in the spleen meridian affecting physical and physiological levels can give rise to the following symptoms:

Abnormal taste, abnormal smell, abnormal uterine bleeding, absence of menstruation, alzheimer's disease, autism, bleeding under the skin, bleeding from the mucous membrane, bruises under the skin, bitter taste in the mouth, cold sores on the lips, carpal tunnel syndrome, coldness of the legs, chronic gastroenteritis, cramps after the first day of menses, depression, diabetes, dizzy spells, dreams that make you tired, emaciated muscles, failing memory, fatigue in general, fatigued limbs, fatigue of the mind, feverishness, fibromyalgia, fluttering of the eyelids, generalized edema, hard lumps in the abdomen, hemophilia, hemorrhoids, hyperglycemia, hypoglycemia, hypertension, inability to make decisions, incontinence of urine, or stool, indigestion, infertility, insomnia usually unable to fall asleep, intractable pain anywhere in the body, intuitive and prophetic behaviors, irregular periods, lack of enthusiasm, lack of interest in anything, lethargy, light headedness, loose stools, nausea, obesity, pain in the great toes, pain and stiffness of the fingers, pallor, pedal edema, prolapse of the uterus, poor memory, prolapse of the bladder, purpura, reduced appetite, sand-like feeling in the eyes, scanty menstrual flow, small, frequent, pencil-like thin stools with undigested food particles, sensation of heaviness in the head, sensation of heaviness in the body, sleep during the day, sluggishness, slowing of the mind, swollen eyelids, swollen lips, swellings or pain with swelling of the toes and feet, fingers and hands, swelling anywhere in the body, stiffness of the tongue, sugar craving, tingling or abnormal sensation in the tip of the fingers and palms, varicose veins, vomiting, and watery eyes.

Energy disturbance in the spleen meridian affecting the cellular level can cause the following:

Worry, concern, anxiety, does not like crowds, easily hurt, gives more importance to self, hopelessness, irritable, keeps feelings inside, lack of confidence, likes loneliness, likes to take revenge, likes to be praised, likes to get constant encouragement — otherwise falls apart, lives through others, low self esteem, obsessive compulsive behavior, over sympathetic to others, restrained, shy, talks to self, timid, and unable to make decisions.

Essential nutrients to strengthen the spleen meridian: Vitamin A, vitamin C, calcium, chromium, protein and sugar.

THE HEART MERIDIAN (HT)

Energy disturbance in the heart meridian affecting physical and physiological levels can give rise to the following symptoms:

Angina-like pains, chest pains, discomfort when reclining, dizziness, dry throat, excessive perspiration, feverishness, headache, heart palpitation, heaviness in the chest, hot palms and soles, insomnia—unable to fall asleep when awakened in the middle of sleep, irritability, mental disorders, nervousness, pain in the eye, pain along the left arm, pain along the scapula, pain and fullness in the chest, poor circulation, shortness of breath, and shoulder pains.

Energy disturbance in the heart meridian affecting the cellular level can cause the following:

Joy, or lack of joy, self-confidence, compassion and love are the emotions of the heart. But when the energy is blocked, one may experience the following: abusive nature, anger, aggression, bad manners, lack of love and compassion, compulsive behaviors, does not trust anyone, does not like to make friends, easily upset, excessive laughing or crying, guilt, hostility, insecurity, lack of emotions, overexcitement, sadness, and type A personality.

Essential nutrients to strengthen the heart meridian: Calcium, vitamin C, vitamin E, fatty acids, selenium, potassium, sodium, iron, and B complex.

THE SMALL INTESTINE MERIDIAN (SI)

Energy disturbance in the small intestine meridian affecting physical and physiological levels can give rise to the following symptoms:

Abdominal pain, abdominal fullness, acne on the upper back, bad breath, bitter taste in the mouth, constipation, diarrhea, distention of lower abdomen, dry stool, frozen shoulder, knee pain, night sweats, numbness of the mouth and tongue, numbness of the back of the shoulder and arm, pain in the neck, pain radiating around the waist, shoulder pain, sore throat, stiff neck, pain along the lateral aspect of the shoulder and arm.

Energy disturbance in the small intestine meridian affecting the cellular level can cause the following:

Insecurity, absent-mindedness, becoming too involved with details, day dreaming, easily annoyed, emotional instability, feeling of abandonment, feeling shy, having a tendency to be introverted and easily hurt, irritability, excessive joy or lack of joy, lacking- confidence, over excitement, paranoia, poor concentration, sadness, sighing, sorrow, suppressing deep sorrow.

Essential nutrients to strengthen the small intestine meridian:

Vitamin B complex, vitamin D, vitamin E, acidophilus, yoghurt, fibers, fatty acids, wheat germ and whole grains.

THE URINARY BLADDER MERIDIAN (UB)

Energy disturbance in the bladder meridian affecting physical and physiological levels can give rise to the following symptoms:

Arthritis of the joints of little finger, bloody urine, burning urination, chills, chronic headaches at the back of the neck, disease of the eye, enuresis, fever, frequent urination, headaches especially at the back of the neck, loss of bladder control, mental disorders, muscle wasting, nasal congestion, pain and discomfort in the lower abdomen, pain in the inner canthus of the eyes, pain behind the knees, pain and stiffness of the back, pain in the fingers and toes, pain in the lateral part of the sole, pain in the lower back, pain along back of the leg and foot, pain in the lateral part of the ankle, pain along the meridian, pain in the little toe, painful urination, retention of urine, sciatic neuralgia, spasm behind the knee, spasms along the posterior part of the thigh and leg, spasms of the calf muscles, stiff neck, weakness in the rectum and rectal muscle.

Energy disturbance in the bladder meridian affecting the cellular level can cause the following:

Fright, sadness, disturbing and impure thoughts, annoyed, fearful, unhappy, frustrated, highly irritable, impatient, inefficient, insecure, reluctant and restless.

Essential nutrients to strengthen the bladder meridian:

Vitamin C, A, E, B complex, especially B_1, calcium, amino acids and trace minerals.

THE KIDNEY MERIDIAN (KI)

Energy disturbance in the kidney meridian affecting physical and physiological levels can give rise to the following symptoms:

Bags under the eyes, blurred vision, burning or painful urination, chronic diarrhea, coldness in the back, cold feet, crave salt, dark circles under the eyes, dryness of the mouth, excessive sleeping, excessive salivation, excessive thirst, facial edema, fatigue, fever with chills, frequent urination, impotence, irritability, light headedness, lower backache, motor impairment, muscular atrophy of the foot, nagging mild asthma, nausea, pain in the sole of the foot, pain in the posterior aspect of the leg or thigh, pain in the ears, poor memory, poor concentration, poor appetite, puffy eyes, ringing in the ears, sore throat, spasms of the ankle and feet, swelling in the legs, swollen ankles and vertigo.

Energy disturbance in the kidney meridian affecting the cellular level can cause the following:

Fear, terror, caution, confused, indecision, seeks attention, unable to express feelings.

Essential nutrients to strengthen the kidney meridian:

Vitamins A, E, B, essential fatty acids, amino acids, sodium chloride, trace minerals, calcium and iron.

THE PERICARDIUM MERIDIAN (PC)

Energy disturbance in the pericardium meridian affecting physical and physiological levels can give rise to the following symptoms:

Chest pain, contracture of the arm or elbow, excessive appetite, fainting spells, flushed face, frozen shoulder, fullness in the chest, heaviness in the chest, hot palms and soles, impaired speech, irritability, nausea, nervousness, pain in the anterior part of the thigh, pain in the eyes, pain in the medial part of the knee, palpitation, restricting movements, sensation of hot or cold, slurred speech, spasms of the elbow, arm and motor impairment of the tongue.

Energy disturbance in the pericardium meridian affecting the cellular level can cause the following:

Shock, hurt, extreme joy, fear of heights, heaviness in the head, heaviness in the chest due to emotional overload, imbalance in sexual energy like never having enough sex, jealousy, light sleep with dreams, manic disorders, in some cases no desire for sex, over-excitement, regret, sexual tension, stubbornness and various phobias.

Essential nutrients to strengthen the pericardium meridian:

Vitamin E, vitamin C, chromium, and trace minerals.

THE TRIPLE WARMER MERIDIAN (TW)

Energy disturbance in the triple warmer meridian affecting physical and physiological levels can give rise to the following symptoms:

Abdominal pain, always feels hungry even after eating a full meal, constipation, deafness, distention, dysuria, edema, enuresis, excessive thirst, excessive hunger, fever in the late evening, frequent urination, hardness and fullness in the lower abdomen, indigestion, pain in the medial part of the knee, pain in the shoulder and upper arm, pain behind the ear, pain in the cheek and jaw, redness in the eye, shoulder pain, swelling and pain in the throat and vertigo.

Energy disturbance in the triple warmer meridian affecting the cellular level can cause the following:

Depression, deprivation, despair, emptiness, excessive emotion, grief, hopelessness and phobias.

Essential nutrients to strengthen the triple warmer meridian:

Iodine, trace minerals, vitamin C, calcium, fluoride and water.

THE GALL BLADDER MERIDIAN (GB)

Energy disturbance in the gall bladder meridian affecting physical and physiological levels can give rise to the following symptoms:

A heavy sensation in the right upper part of the abdomen, abdominal bloating, alternating fever and chills, ashen complexion, bitter taste in the mouth, burping after meals, chills, deafness, dizziness, fever, headaches on the sides of the head, heartburn after fatty foods, hyperacidity, moving arthritis, pain in the jaw, nausea with fried foods, pain in the eye, pain in the hip, pain and cramps along the anterolateral wall, poor digestion of fats, sciatic neuralgia, sighing, stroke-like condition, swelling in the submaxillary region, tremors, twitching, vision disturbances, vomiting and yellowish complexion.

Energy disturbance in the gall bladder meridian affecting the cellular level can cause the following:

Gall bladder is associated with control issues, rage, aggression, complaining all the time, fearful, finding faults with others and unhappiness.

Essential nutrients to strengthen the gall bladder meridian:

Vitamin A, apples, lemon, calcium, linoleic acids and oleic acids (for example, pine nuts, olive oil).

THE LIVER MERIDIAN (LIV)

Energy disturbance in the liver meridian affecting physical and physiological levels can give rise to the following symptoms:

Abdominal pain, blurred vision, dark urine, dizziness, enuresis, excessive bright colored bleeding during menses, feeling of some obstruction in the throat, fever, hard lumps in the upper abdomen, headache at the top of the head, hernia, hemiplegia, irregular menses, jaundice, loose stools, pain in the intercostal region, pain in the breasts, pain in the lower abdomen, paraplegia, PMS, reproductive organ disturbances, retention of urine, seizures, spasms in the extremities, stroke-like condition, tinnitus, vertigo, and vomiting.

Energy disturbance in the liver meridian affecting the cellular level can cause the following:

Anger, irritability, aggression, assertion, rage, shouting, talking loud and type A personality.

Essential nutrients to strengthen the liver meridian: Beets, green vegetables, vitamin A, trace minerals and unsaturated fatty acids.

THE GOVERNING VESSEL MERIDIAN

Energy disturbance in the governing vessel meridian affecting physical, physiological and psychological levels can give rise to the following symptoms:

This channel supplies the brain and spinal region and intersects the liver channel at the vertex. Obstruction of its Chi may result in symptoms such as stiffness and pain along the spinal column. Deficient Chi in the channel may produce a heavy sensation in the head, vertigo and shaking. Energy blockages in this meridian (which passes through the brain) may be responsible for certain mental disorders. Febrile diseases are commonly associated with the governing vessel channel and because one branch of the channel ascends through the abdomen, when the channel is unbalanced, its Chi rushes upward toward the heart. Symptoms such as colic, constipation, enuresis, hemorrhoids and functional infertility may result.

THE CONCEPTION VESSEL MERIDIAN (CV, REN)

Energy disturbance in the conception vessel meridian affecting physical, physiological and psychological levels can give rise to the following symptoms:

The conception vessel channel is the confluence of the Yin channels. Therefore, abnormality along the conception vessel channel will appear principally in pathological symptoms of the Yin channels, especially symptoms associated with the liver and kidneys. Its function is closely related with pregnancy and, therefore, has intimate links with the kidneys and uterus. If its Chi is deficient, infertility or other disorders of the urogenital system may result. Leukorrhea, irregular menstruation, colic, etc., are associated with the conception vessel channel.

Any allergen can cause blockage in one or more meridians at the same time. If it is causing blockages in only one meridian, the patient may demonstrate symptoms related to that particular meridian. The intensity of the symptoms will depend on the severity of the blockage. The patient may suffer from one symptom, many symptoms or all the symptoms of this meridian. Sometimes, a patient can have many meridians blocked at the same time. In such cases, the patient may demonstrate a variety of symptoms, one symptom from each meridian or many symptoms from certain meridians and one or two from other meridians. Some patients with blockage in one meridian can demonstrate just one symptom from the list, but may be with great intensity.

Some people, even though they have disturbances in all meridians, may not show any symptoms. Such patients might have a better immune system than others. Variations with all these possibilities make diagnosis difficult in some cases.

CHAPTER 6

Muscle Response Testing

Muscle response testing is one of the tools used by kinesiologists to test the kinetic imbalances in the body. The same muscle response testing can also be used in detecting allergens that cause allergic reactions and allergy-based disorders in the body.

Muscle response testing has been practiced in this country since 1964. It was originated by Dr. George Goodheart and his associates. Dr. John F. Thie advocates this method through the "Touch For Health" Foundation in Malibu, California. Interested readers can write to "Touch For Health" Foundation for information and books on the subject.

When the allergen's incompatible electromagnetic energy comes close to a person's energy field, repulsion takes place. Without recognizing this repulsive action, we frequently go near allergens (whether they are foods, drinks, chemicals, environmental substances, animals or humans) and interact with their energies. This energy disturbance produces energy blockages in the energy meridians, creating disorganization in body functioning, giving rise to various types of allergic reactions and diseases.

To prevent the allergen from causing further disarray after producing the initial blockage, the brain sends messages to every cell of the body to reject the presence of the allergen. This rejection will appear as repulsion, and this repulsion can be seen as different physical, physiological and psychological symptoms in the person, like weak limbs, tiredness, aches, pains, insomnia, constipation, anger, depression and many other such unpleasant symptoms.

Your body has a way of telling you when you are in trouble. When you go near allergens, your brain will begin to produce various symptoms in your body in varying degrees, such as: an itchy throat, watery eyes, sneezing attacks, coughing spells, unexplained pain anywhere in the body, yawning, sudden tiredness, etc. If you learn to understand your brain and its clues closely you may be able to avoid many unpleasant events in your life, including many serious health disorders. Muscle response testing is a good tool that can be used successfully to identify the allergens. In this muscle response testing procedure, you will compare the strength of a strong muscle in your body in the presence and absence of a suspected allergen. If a previously strong muscle tests weak in the presence of a substance, the substance is an allergen. If the substance was not able to elicit a weakness in the previously strong muscle, then the substance is not an allergen. NAET specialists use muscle response testing to identify the presence of allergens around you.

Muscle Response Testing (MRT)
(See illustrations of MRT on the following pages.)

Muscle response testing can be performed in the following ways:

1. Standard muscle response testing can be done in standing, sitting or lying positions. You need two people to do this test: the person who is testing, the "tester," and the person being tested, the "subject."

2.	The oval ring test and finger on finger test can be used in testing yourself. Oval ring test can also be used in testing a physically strong person. To test another person using Oval ring testing requires two persons, as in standard muscle response testing.

3.	Surrogate testing can be used in testing an infant, an invalid, a very strong or a very weak person, an animal, a plant or a tree. In this case, the surrogate's muscle is tested by the tester, and

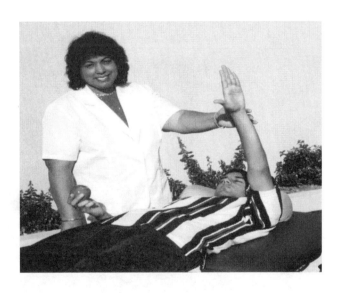

Fig. 6-1
Standard MRT

the subject maintains skin-to-skin contact with the surrogate while being tested and/or treated. The surrogate is not affected by the testing or treatment.

Standard Muscle Response Testing

Two people are required to perform standard muscle response testing. The subject can be tested lying down, standing or sitting. The lying-down position is the most convenient for both tester and subject. It also achieves more accurate results.

Step 1: The subject lies on a firm surface with one arm raised (left arm in the picture below) 45-90 degrees to the body with

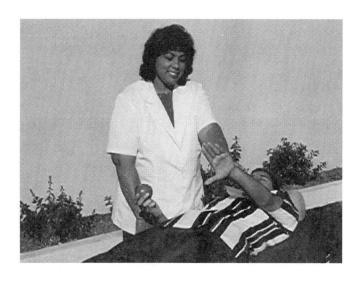

Fig. 6-2
MRT with an Allergen

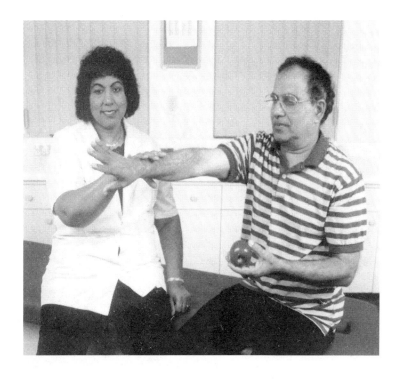

Fig. 6-3
MRT with Allergen in Sitting Position

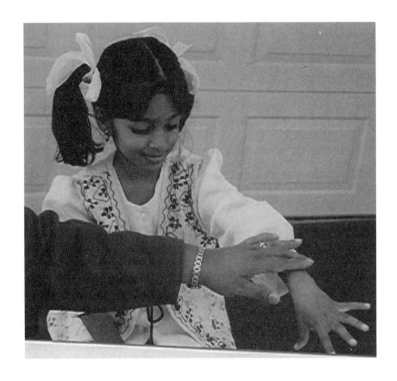

Fig. 6-4
MRT with Allergen in Standing Position

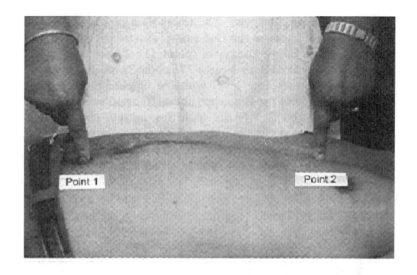

Fig. 6-5
Balancing the Body

the palm facing outward and the thumb facing toward the big toe.

Step 2:   The tester stands at the subject's (right) side. The subject's right arm is kept to his/her side with the palm either kept open to the air, or in a loose fist. The fingers should not touch any material, fabric or any part of the table the arm is resting on. This can give wrong test results. The left arm of the subject is raised 45-90 degrees to the body. The tester's left palm is contacting the subject's left wrist (Figure 6-1).

Step 3:   The tester, using the left arm, tries to push down on the subject's raised left arm toward the subject's left big toe. The subject resists the push with the arm muscle. The test muscle is called an "indicator muscle or predetermined muscle" or PDM for short. The PDM remains strong if the subject is well balanced at the time of testing. It is essential to test a strong PDM to get accurate results. Either the subject is not balanced, or the tester is performing the test improperly if the muscle or raised arm is weak and gives way under pressure without the presence of an allergen. For example, the tester might be trying to overpower the subject. The subject does not need to gather up strength from other muscles in the body to resist the tester. Only five to ten pounds of pressure needs to be applied on the muscle, for three to five seconds. The tester will feel a sensation of "lock" at the arm if he/she is testing the arm properly and if the subject is resisting the push appropriately. If the muscle tests weak, the tester will be able to judge the difference with that small amount of pressure (5-10 lbs of pressure) he/she is applying. It may sound very easy, but much practice is needed to learn the procedure properly. If you cannot test effectively the first few times, there is no need to get frustrated. Please remember that practice makes perfect.

Step 4: If the indicator muscle remains strong when tested without the presence of an allergen, —a sign that the subject is found to be balanced—then the tester should put the suspected allergen into the palm of the subject's resting hand. The sensory receptors, on the tips of the fingers, are extremely sensitive in recognizing allergens. When the subject's fingertips touch the allergen, the sensory receptors from the fingertips sense the charges of the allergen and relay the message to the brain. The fingertips have specialized sensory receptors that can send messages to the brain and receive the replies from the brain in a nanosecond. If the charges are compatible to the body, the indicator muscle will remain strong. If the charges are incompatible, the strong PDM will go weak. This tells you that you are allergic (sensitive) to the item.

Step 5: This step is useful in balancing the patient if he/she is found to be weak on the initial testing without the presence of an allergen. You need to make the patient's test muscle strong before you can test and compare the strength of the muscle with and without the allergen. The tester places his/her fingertips of one hand at "point 1" on the midline of the subject, about one and a half inches below the navel at the conception vessel "6"(see below). The other hand is placed on conception vessel "17" (point 2), in the center of the chest on the midline, level with the nipple line. The tester massages these two points clockwise gently and simultaneously with the fingertips about 20 or 30 seconds, then repeats steps 2 and 3. If the indicator muscle tests strong, continue on to step 4. If the indicator muscle tests weak again, repeat this procedure several times. It is very unlikely that any person will remain weak after repeating this procedure two to three times.

Point 1: Name of the point: Sea of Energy, (conception vessel 6)
Location: One and a half inches below the navel, on the midline. This is where the energy of the body is stored in abundance. When the body senses any danger around its energy field or when the body experiences energy blockages, the energy supply is cut short and stored here. If you massage clockwise on this energy reservoir point, the energy will flow out of the storage towards the energy channels and make the weak area strong again.

Point 2: Name of the point: Dominating Energy, (Conception vessel 17)

Location: In the center of the chest on the midline of the body, level with the fourth intercostal space. This is the energy dispenser unit. This is the point that controls and regulates the energy circulation, or Chi, in the body. When the energy rises from the *Sea of Energy*, it flows straight to the *Dominating Energy* point. From here, the energy is dispersed to different meridians, organs, tissues and cells as needed to help remove the energy blockages. It does this by forcing energy circulation from inside out. During this forced energy circulation, the blockages are pushed out of the body, balancing the body's state. You feel this through the strength of the indicator muscle.

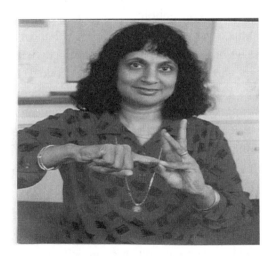

Fig. 6-6
"O" Ring Test

Oval Ring, or 'O' Ring Test

The oval ring test can be used in self-testing. This can also be used to test a subject if the subject is physically very strong with a strong arm and the tester is a physically weak person.

Step 1: The tester makes an "O" shape by opposing the little finger and thumb on the same hand. Then, with the index finger of the other hand, he/she tries to separate the "O" ring against pressure. If the little finger and thumb separates easily, test the ring finger and thumb. It should remain strong. If that also goes weak with medium pressure, use the middle finger and thumb. It should remain strong. Find a finger-thumb combination that can resist the pressure of the index finger of the other hand. Use that finger-thumb combination as the test muscle. If you can't find any strong combination, you need to balance the body using step-5 from Standard MRT.

Step 2: If the "O" ring remains inseparable and fairly strong, hold the allergen in the other hand, by the fingertips, and perform step 1 again. If the "O" ring separates easily, the

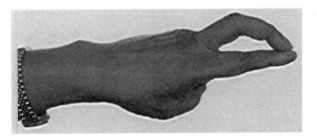

Fig. 6-7
Finger on Finger Test

person is allergic to the substance he/she is touching. If the "O" ring remains strong, the substance is not an allergen.

This can also be done through another person. The person whose fingers are being tested will be considered a surrogate.

The Finger-on-finger Test

The finger-on-finger test (Figure 6-7) is another way to test yourself. The strength of the interphalangeal muscles of two fingers of one hand is used here to test and compare the strength while holding an allergen. The middle finger is pushed down by the index finger or the index finger is pushed down by the middle finger of the same hand, in the absence and presence of the allergen in the other hand. This technique also needs much practice.

Step 1: The tester places the pad of the index finger at the back of the middle finger of the same hand. The middle finger is pushed down, using the index finger of the same hand. If the middle finger could resist the push by the index finger, then the person is balanced. If the person is not balanced, please balance using the same step-5 from standard MRT. When the person is balanced, go to the next step.

Step 2: Then the tester holds the allergen in one hand. Next he/she again places the pad of the index finger at the back of the middle finger of the same hand. The middle finger is pushed down, using the index finger of the same hand. The item you are holding is an allergen if the middle finger goes down easily while pushing with the index finger in the presence of the item.

Muscle response testing is one of the most reliable methods of allergy testing, if done properly. It needs much practice to get accurate results. Follow the tips given in the next page to master muscle response testing to perfection.

After considerable practice, some people are able to test themselves very efficiently using these methods. When they complete 30 to 40 NAET treatments successfully with an NAET specialist, they will be about 70-80 percent free of their allergies. But, in order to have freedom to live in this chemically polluted world, it is very important for allergic people to learn some form of self-testing technique that enables them to screen out possible allergens from their daily life before contacting them. When the patients learn the NAET testing techniques described in this Chapter, they will be able to test them and identify the allergens before they expose themselves to them. It takes considerable amount of practice. When it is identified it is easy to avoid. This will help them to prevent unexpected allergic reactions. This will also provide them confidence, freedom to eat, freedom to go to places, and freedom to live again.

Hundreds of new allergens are thrown into the world daily by non-allergic people who do not understand the predicament of the allergic population. If you want to live in this world looking and feeling normal among normal people, side by side with the allergens, you need to learn how to test on your own. You will not be totally free from allergies until you learn to test accurately. It takes many hours (months in some cases) of practice. But do not get discouraged. I have given enough information on testing methods here. You need to spend time and practice until you reach perfection.

A Tip to Master Self-Testing

Step 1:   Find two items, or two groups of items (collect a few samples of known allergens for you). Then collect another group that you are not allergic to. Let's assume that you are allergic to the group A and not allergic to group B in the list.

Allergen Practice List For Self-Testing

Group A	Group B
(Non-allergic items)	(allergic items)
apple	banana
book	peanut
polyester	Pen
plastic bag	orange
car key	computer key board
milk	coffee
cucumber	chicken
corn	green pepper
potato	potato
plastic bag	jello-pudding

Table 6-1

Step 2: Hold the samples from group A one at a time in one hand and test with the other hand, using either "O" ring testing or finger on finger testing. The ring easily breaks in the case of "O" ring testing or the interphalangeal muscle weakens easily if you are using finger-on-finger testing. The same way, test each item from group B one by one. The "O" ring remains strong and the middle finger will not be pushed down by the index finger when you test items from the non-allergic group.Rub your hands together or wash your hands between touching different testing samples.

Step 3: When you test the allergic items, if the muscle doesn't go weak, make it happen intentionally for the first few times.

Now, hold the items from non-allergic group and do the same test. This time, the ring doesn't break. Practice this procedure for awhile. Rub your hands together for 30 seconds between changing the test samples to interrupt the energy at the fingertips of the previous sample.

Practice this every day. Eventually, your subconscious mind will be able to recognize the strength of the allergen just by touching it with your fingertips. When you master this procedure, you can test anything around you. Table 6-1 is an example of gathering a practice list of commonly seen allergens. You can create your own practice list of allergens and non-allergens.

Surrogate Testing

This method can be very useful to test and determine the allergies of an infant, a child, an invalid or disabled person, an unconscious person, an extremely strong, or very weak person, because they do not have conclusive muscle strength to perform an allergy test. You can also use this method to test an animal, a plant, or a tree.

The surrogate's muscle is tested by the tester. It is very important to remember to maintain skin-to-skin contact between the surrogate and the subject during the procedure. If you maintain the skin-to-skin contact, then the surrogate will not receive the results of the testing and treatment. If you break the skin-to-skin contact then the surrogate will get part of the result while the contact was off.

NAET treatments can be administered through the surrogate very effectively without causing any interference to the surrogate's energy. The testing or treatment does not affect the surrogate as long as the subject maintains uninterrupted skin-to-skin contact with him/her.

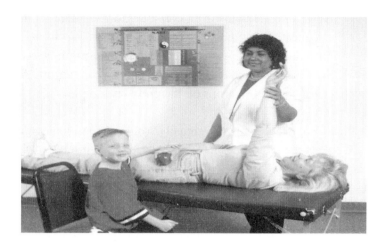

Fig. 6-8
Testing through a Surrogate

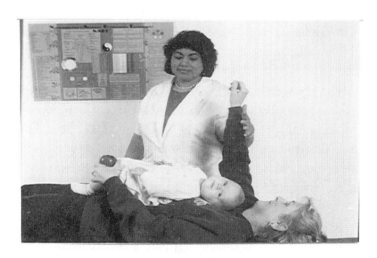

Fig. 6-9
Testing an Infant

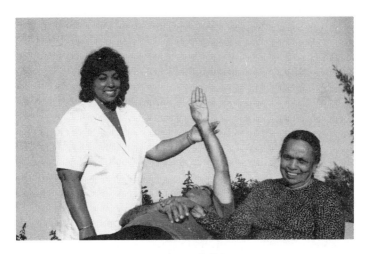

Fig. 6-10
Testing for Person to Person allergy

Testing for Person to Person Allergy

You can test an allergy to anything around you using muscle response testing. You can test your allergy to your children, spouse, friends, and other family members using this method. When you test for allergies to another person, the person-A lies down and touches person-B (the suspected allergen). The tester pushes the arm of person-A as in steps 2 and 3. If person-A is allergic to person-B, the indicator muscle goes weak. If the person-A is not allergic to person-B, the indicator muscle remains strong.

If people are allergic to each other (husband and wife, mother and child, father and son, patient and doctor, etc.), the allergy can affect a person in various ways. Husband and wife might fight all the time or if they do not have the nature to fight, their health can be affected. The same things can happen among other family members too. It is important to test the family members and other immediate associates for person-to-person allergy and, if found, family members and/or associates should be treated for each other to obtain health, wealth and happiness.

Testing Owner's Allergy to an Animal

You can check your allergy to your pets, and the pet's allergy towards you using the same method.

The owner's muscle is tested by the tester while the owner maintains the fingertip-contact on the skin of the pet with the free hand. It is very important to remember to maintain skin-to-skin contact between the owner and the pet.

Procedure:

Step :   The owner holds the pet (the allergen) with the finger-tips resting on the animal's body while the tester pushes on the raised hand of the owner. If the MRT is weak, the owner is allergic to the pet. The owner can get treated for the animal by maintaining the contact on its body while the doctor is administering the treatment.

Treating Pet's Allergy towards Substances

You can test your pet's allergy towards other substances using the same method. You can treat the pets through a surrogate for their allergy to the substances. Pets could be found to be allergic to their daily foods, drinks, water, toys, living environment, sleeping rug or mat, vitamins, drugs, vaccination, insects, collar, litter-box, etc.

Procedure:

Surrogate holds the suspected allergen in his/her hand and touches the pet with the fingers while the tester is testing with MRT.

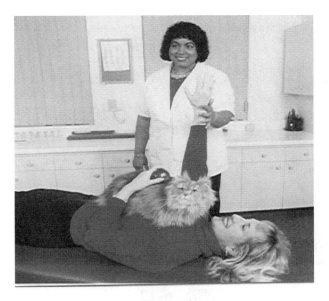

Fig. 6-11
Testing a Pet's Allergy

If the MRT is weak, the pet is allergic to the item. You can treat the animal through the surrogate as one would treat an infant.

Treating the Pet's Allergy Towards the Owner

Step 1: In this case the owner will be the surrogate. The owner's muscle is tested by the tester while the owner maintains skin-to-skin contact on the pet with the free hand. It is very important to remember to maintain skin-to-skin contact between the owner and the pet.

Step 2: The owner holds the pet and make the animal's paw touch the body of the owner. The tester pushes on the raised arm of the owner while the animal's paw is resting on the owner's other arm. If the MRT is weak, the pet is allergic to the owner. Treat the pet through surrogate by maintain-

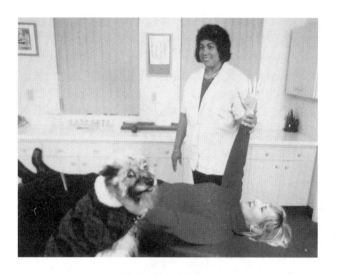

Fig. 6-12
Testing Owner's Allergy to Pet

ing the same contact. The owner touches the pet while doing MRT. If the MRT goes weak, then the owner is allergic to the pet. Then the owner should hold the pet by maintaining contact on the body, while the doctor is administering the treatment.

CHAPTER 7

Living with Allergies

We have seen how allergies can interfere with our lives, how allergies can complicate our existence and take the pleasure out of living. You will be amazed to find that many of the medical problems you suffer may have allergies as their origins. Using the methods described in Chapter 6, you can learn to test your allergies and discover the causes of most of your common illnesses or "incurable" disorders.

If you learn the testing procedures and practice at home, it won't be long before you find out that most of your health problems (or your loved one's) have their roots in your daily diets, or clothes, even in the vitamins you were using which you thought were helping you to live healthy and well.

How surprised you will be when you discover (for example) that:

Your 20-year-old eczema was due to an allergy to eggs and aggravated by eating eggs and chicken products or due to dried beans (proteins) taken to supplement your diet with enough protein?

An allergy to your soft, expensive feather pillow was causing your chronic sinusitis.

Your incurable osteoporosis was due to an allergy to calcium and aggravated by drinking three glasses of milk every day to supplement natural calcium.

Your joint pains and arthritis were due to an allergy to citrus fruits and aggravated by drinking a glass of grapefruit juice for breakfast.

Your daily, nagging migraines were due to an allergy to whole wheat and aggravated by eating a dry slice of whole wheat bread for breakfast.

The fatigue you experience every afternoon was contributed by an allergy to chocolate and aggravated by the Snickers bar you eat every day after lunch to feed that sweet tooth.

Your 15-year-old lower backache was due to an allergy to iron, and aggravated by eating a juicy hamburger twice a week to supplement iron and vitamin B_{12}.

The rough, scaly skin was actually due to an allergy to vitamin A and aggravated by eating carrots for snacks daily to supplement your vitamin A requirement to maintain good eyesight and soft skin texture.

Your bad breath, brittle nails, low energy, quick temper were contributed by an allergy to trace minerals chromium and zinc.

Your abdominal bloating around your menstrual cycle was due to an allergy to the salt you add when you cook meals.

Your child's chronic bronchitis was probably due to an allergy to that one glass of orange juice he drinks every morning.

Your child's hyperactivity and poor attention span were caused by an allergy to the coloring pencils and crayons he uses to color in the school every day.

Your child's Dr. Jekyll and Mr. Hyde-like behavior was caused by an allergy to the whole wheat cereal and low fat milk he eats at breakfast.

Your child's frequent colds and sore throat were due to an allergy to the city water he drinks in school.

Your husband's two-month-old walking pneumonia was due to an allergy to the yoghurt he eats daily for lunch at work.

Your irritating yeast-like infection was due to the allergy to the toilet paper you use daily.

The shocking fact is that if one evaluates carefully, 90% of human health disorders have some form of allergy involvement. These allergies can make you sick or at least put you "under the weather." If you learn how to test and find your allergies, if you learn how to find the cause of your illnesses before they cripple you, you could avoid mental agony. Now you have a way to do just that. You can test and find your allergies within the privacy of your own home, without going through expensive and extensive laboratory tests. (Caution: If you are suffering from a major sickness, please see your doctor or appropriate specialist immediately and get evaluated first). Just by avoiding the allergens from your life, you will be able to live peacefully. If you must use the products, please see a practitioner who is trained in NAET. If you take time to read this book, you will understand how to help yourself with mild to moderate allergies, because some self-help tips are given in Chapter 8. If you are one with many allergies, with severe symptoms, please consult an NAET specialist right away to get a few NAET treatments before you try self-help procedures. For complicated problems, you need to consult an appropriate specialist.

Every one should be tested and treated for all NAET Basic allergen groups, these are the very basic treatments. NAET basic treatments include the basic essentials of life, the most commonly used food and enzymes from everyday life. If one is allergic to all the essential nutrients, he/she can become reactive to everything else around him/her. By eliminating the allergies to the essential nutrients, one's immunity will improve or maintain at a very high level, with the result, one may not get other allergies or allergy based illnesses as often as others who have not had the NAET Basic treatments.

But it might help the NAET patient to learn certain rules before he/she begins the treatment.

Instructions to the NAET Patient Before Beginning Treatment

1. Patients should be encouraged to read *Say Good-bye To Illness* before they begin the NAET treatments. Doctor should explain the treatment procedure to the patient before beginning the treatment.

2. If you have any laboratory reports from previous doctor, please bring them with you.

3. Please do not wear any perfume, perfumed powder, strong smelling deodorant, hair spray, or after shave, eat strong smelling herbs like raw garlic, etc., when you come to the clinic for treatments. Do not bring any little children or pets to the clinic when you come for the treatment. No one should sit or stand in the room when the doctor is testing or treating the patient. The presence of a third person or animal can negate your treatment if the third person is standing in your energy field while you get the NAET treatment.

4. There is no smoking allowed in (or around) the office. Please do not wear clothes that smell like smoke or paint. Other patients could react to these smells.

5. Please wash your hands before and after the treatment. After the treatment, instead of washing the hands, vigorous rubbing of the hands for 30 seconds will be sufficient.

6. Do not exercise for 6 hours after the treatment.

7. Avoid exposure to extreme hot or cold temperature after the treatment.

8. Please take a shower before you come in for a treatment, and wear freshly washed clothes to avoid smell of herbs, spices, perspiration, etc. from your body or clothes. This can cause irritation and reactions in other allergic patients.

9. Do not bathe or shower until 6 hours after the treatment.

10. Do not eat or chew gum or candy during treatment.

11. After each NAET treatment, you are required to wait in the office for 20 minutes. Do not cross your hands or feet during the first 20 minutes after the treatment.

12. Do not read or touch other objects during the 20 minutes following the treatment because contact with other substances during this period could cause your treatment to fail.

13. Wear minimum or no jewelry when you come for a treatment. Avoid wearing large crystals or large diamonds.

14. For best results, after each treatment, the treated allergen must be avoided for 25 hours or more. The patients who follows 25-hour avoidance get the best result from NAET. During 25 hours, the body goes through natural detoxification. Often these patients do not require to go through other detoxification procedures. If you need more hours of waiting period after the treatment, your NAET specialist can check the time and inform you after each treatment. Remember to check with your doctor for the item you treated, after 25 hours, and at least within one week to make sure you have completed the treatment. If you did not complete the treatment, your symptoms due to the incomplete treatment may continue for a long time, sometimes for weeks. Eventually the symptoms will wear off if you did not repeat the treatment for the unfinished allergen.

If you are in the doctor's office for any acute reaction, your doctor (practitioner) may treat you for the allergen causing the acute reaction. That is the only time a true NAET doctor will treat out of the given order.

If your practitioner is not confident to treat your acute problem using NAET, please go to the nearest emergency room or if you are very sick to travel, please call 911 immediately.

15. To insure maximum progress with your treatments maintain your own treatment and food diary in the NAET guide book at the section for record keeping. If you need help to record your treatments, please ask your practitioner.

16. You may need to take extra precaution while you get treated for environmental substances: (mineral mix, metals, water, leather, formaldehyde, fabric, wood, mold, mercury, newspaper, marker ink, chemicals, flowers, perfume, etc.). Apart from staying away from the item, you may also need

to wear mask, gloves, socks and shoes even to bed, full gowns, scarf, earplugs, covering your head, ear, and forehead, etc., for 25 hours following treatment.

17. Always eat before you come for the treatment. You should not take NAET treatments and acupuncture when you are hungry. If you have a long wait in your doctor's office, please bring a snack with you and eat it just before the treatment

18. Do not eat heavy meals after the NAET treatments.

19. Drink a glass of water before the treatment. Energy moves better in a well hydrated body. Drink lots of water (4-6 glasses/day) after each NAET treatments to help flush out the toxins produced during the treatment.

20. Please do not stop any other treatment you are on: medication, therapy, chiropractic treatments, acupuncture, massages, etc. It is good for your body to have a general body massage before the NAET or 6 hours after the NAET treatments. Massages can help to improve the energy flow through the energy pathways. If you are taking lots of vitamins and herbs, or any particular drug, you may continue them as before if you think that they are helping you. But when you get treated for the food containing a particular vitamin, herb, or substance, at certain times you may be asked to stop it for 25 hours following that particular treatment or use a substitute.

21. NAET treatment will not interfere with any other treatment. In fact, if you can keep your body free of toxin accumulation (stool softeners, laxatives, to prevent constipation, and colonics or high enemas once or twice a month to eliminate the toxic build up), and keeping your symptoms under control with whatever method you are using, NAET treatment will be a lot easier.

22. NAET Treatments for allergens are not advisable when the patient is extremely tired, worked long hours, or worked night shift without any rest, extremely hungry, or had an emotional trauma within a few hours.

23. Teach your patient how to test their allergies at home for their daily usable items and self-treatment to handle the possible emergencies.

24. If the patient is having difficult time to pass an allergen, teach them to massage general balancing points every two hours while awake, by thinking about the sample.

25. For female patients: Treatments are not advisable during the first three days of menstrual cycle.

26. Advise the patient to take a break from the treatment after completing every items.

NAET Basic Allergens

1. BBF (Autonomic nervous system balance)

2. Egg mix (Proteins)

3. Calcium mix

4. Vitamin C mix

5. B complex

6. Sugar mix

7. Iron mix

8. Vitamin A mix

9. Minerals, water, drinking water, city water

10. Salt Mix

11. Grains

12. Yeast mix, yogurt and whey

13. Stomach acid

14. Digestive enzymes or Base

15. Hormones

NAET Classic Allergens

The NAET Classic Allergens include the 15 NAET Basic Allergens groups and 40 other major allergen groups. There are 55 major groups of allergens in the NAET classic allergens. The preferred order of treatments is given below. About 80 percent of one's allergic reactions towards substances will diminish if one clears 100 percent on all these allergens.

16. Artificial sweeteners

17. Coffee, chocolate and caffeine

18. Spice mix 1 & 2

19. Vegetable fat & animal fat

20. Nut mix-1 & nut mix-2

21. Fish and Shell fish

22. Amino acids 1 & 2

23. Whiten-all

24. Turkey/serotonin

25 Fluoride

26. Gum mix

27. Dried bean mix

28. Alcohol

29. Gelatin

30. Vitamin D

31. Vitamin E

32. Vitamin F (fatty acids)

33. Vitamin T (thymus)

34. R.N.A. & D.N.A.

35 Food coloring/food additives

36. Starch mix (Carbohydrates)

37. Nightshade vegetables/vegetable mix

38. Virus mix

39. Bacteria Mix

40. Parasites

41. Chemicals (soap, detergent, etc.)

42. Pollens

43. Grasses/weeds

44. Formaldehyde

45. Latex/plastics

46. Crude oil/Synthetic materials, etc.

47. Animal epithelial/dander

48. Smoking/nicotine

49. Dust/ dust mites

50. Perfume mix/ flowers

51. Immunizations/vaccinations/ drugs

52. Organs or tissues (a particular part of the body that is involved with the disease process. For example: lung, liver, hypothalamus, etc.)

53. Neuro-transmitters

54. Pesticides

55. Heavy metals

Treatment by Priority

After completing the basic 15, your NAET practitioner will evaluate your progress and if needed plan your treatment by priority to help with your immediate health problem, for example: Treat allergen that will help with P.M.S., learning disability, dyslexia, ADHD, autism, migraine headaches, asthma, etc. After the basic fifteen, the rest of the classic NAET allergen groups can be rearranged to help with the immediate problem. This is called "treatment by priority."

What is treatment by priority? Let us look at some examples:

- If your major complaint was "asthma," after completing basic 15, if your asthma is still not under control, your NAET practitioner will begin treating specific allergens related to triggering asthma. For example: Dust mix, grass-pollens, cold (ice cube), etc.

- If you suffer from chemical sensitivities, soon after you complete the basic 15, your practitioner will treat you for formaldehyde, house-cleaning chemicals, etc.

- If your child has ADHD or autism, after completion of basic 15, your NAET practitioner will treat for vaccinations, drugs taken in the past, or neurotransmitters.

All these individual treatment will work better after clearing allergies for essential nutrients— that is the NAET Basic 15 Allergens.

If you see your NAET practitioner for any acute allergic attacks (Migraine, asthma, sudden pain somewhere in the body, etc.), if your practitioner is confident to treat an acute symptom, he/she may treat an allergen or a group of allergens out of the preferred order. If the practitioner is not experienced or not confident to treat an acute problem like asthma please call emergency help by calling 911 in United States. When the acute symptom gets resolved, you can begin the treatment for the first allergen from the basic-15 list starting from the following visit. NAET treatments can give quicker and lasting relief if done properly. If it is not done properly, you may not get the expected results. After about 15 visits, if you don't see any improvement in your condition, you and your practitioner should get together and evaluate the situation.

CHAPTER 8

NAET Self-Help

The purpose of this book is not to train a lay person in medical procedures.The real purpose of this book is to inform people about NAET allergy elimination treatment, so that needy patients can learn about the availability of such a treatment and, if interested, can locate the appropriate medical practitioners with proper NAET training to help eliminate their allergies.

Information regarding a few important acupressure points, and NAET energy balancing points are described in the following pages. These points and techniques, when used properly according to the accompanying instructions, might help to reduce or control your presenting acute allergic symptoms. If used properly, these points can be helpful in emergency situations.

A few self-help energy balancing applications are also discussed in this chapter, with illustrations. These balancing techniques are safe to use on people at any age and in any condition. These procedures can be safely used in balancing animals too. When one maintains energy in a balanced state, the body may not experience any illness or adverse reactions. Just by balancing the body regularly, by maintaining a balanced state, many people have reported that they were able to keep their allergic reactions under control. Some have reported reduction in their allergy-related other health conditions as well.

But again I would like to make the reader aware that these are only energy balancing techniques and should not be confused with actual NAET treatment procedures done with a trained NAET specialist. These balancing techniques will not replace the need for a trained practitioner. These techniques alone are not sufficient to permanently eliminate your allergies. These procedures, when used properly as described in the following pages, will: help to improve overall health, reduce allergies and allergic reactions, help with allergy-related health problems, but <u>will not eliminate your allergies</u>.

Testing

In Chapter 6, you learned to test and find your allergies using MRT. You have learned to test and identify allergens in general. If you want to be healthy, you are urged to practice these testing techniques and make a habit of testing everything you suspect before exposing yourself to them. When you identify your allergens, you may be able to avoid them easily.

I spent countless hours testing, determining, researching, and trying out all my NAET discoveries on hundreds of people before I began sharing them with others. I was a desperate patient myself sometime ago. I was told to learn to live with my chronic pains for the rest of my life. So I understand the pain of living with sickness and feeling trapped.

Now, we have a simple, safe, inexpensive, uncomplicated procedure to test allergies and allergy-related disorders with maximum accuracy.

You can test any type of allergen in this fashion. I am going to list a few commonly encountered, unsuspected, allergens below. When I tell someone to test each and every item before using, most people do not understand that one could be allergic to a vast number of everyday items around them. Most people, including some practitioners, miss unsuspected hidden allergens. These people continue to suffer from various health problems and eventually, when their finances, spirits, motivation and hopes get exhausted, join the club of "Victims of Incurable Disorders."

Treatment

We treat many acute pains using NAET. But soon after the acute pain or symptoms are treated, we encourage our patients to return to the clinic to begin NAET basic treatments. NAET basic treatments are one's basic essentials for survival. Basic essentials are described in Chapter 7. When the patients are treated for basic essentials, they improve their immune system and maintain a good immune system over the years. Allergies and allergy-related diseases tend not to manifest in people with good immune system.

We have found from our experience that patients who get treated just for acute symptoms or presenting symptoms like headaches, backaches, arthritis, abdominal pains, etc., on the initial couple of visits and never return for NAET basic essentials, continue to get various other sicknesses throughout their lives. Because of this we encourage you to complete NAET basic 15 before you stop treatments so that you will not continue to get more unrelated sicknesses in the future.

Commonly Seen Allergens Around You

After-shave lotion, razor-blades
Animals, their epithelial and dander
Bed, bed linen, bed sheet, comforter, and blanket
Books, papers, pens and pencils
Carpets and drapes
Ceramic cups and tiles on the floor

Chemicals, soap, and detergents
Child's school work materials
Clothing, bath towels and other fabrics
Colored clothes (people can be allergic to different colors)
Coloring books
Computer screen, keyboard, desk, and chair
Cooking dishes
Dishwashing soaps and scrubbers
Drinking water and tap water
Drinks
Eating utensils like plates, spoons, fork
Fruits and vegetables
Night gowns, Pajamas
Grains and breads
Hair shampoo, hair conditioner and body lotions
Housecleaning products
Latex gloves and office products
Leaves, weeds, grass, and flowers
Lipstick and other cosmetics
Oils, and other food items
Newspaper and ink
Pillow and pillow case
Salt and sugar
Toothbrush, toothpaste, mouthwash, dental floss
Toothpick, Q-tips, other hygienic materials
Toys, stuffed animals
Vitamins and drugs
Work materials

NAET Self-Testing Procedure #1
Hold, Sit and Test

This is the most simple allergy testing procedure (also read Chapter 4). We teach this to our patients during patient-education class. This is very simple and our young patients love it. Children are thrilled by this procedure. They test secretly for their food, cookies, drinks, clothes, etc., before the parents get to test them with MRT.

Materials Needed:

1. A sample holder (thin glass jar, test tube, or a baby food jar with a lid can serve as a sample-holder).

2. Samples of the suspected allergens.

All perishable items, liquids, foods, should be placed inside the jar, then the lid should be closed tightly so that the smell will not bother the patient. If it is a piece of fabric, toy, etc., it can be held in the hand. Severe allergens like pesticides, perfume, chemicals, other toxic products should only be self-tested by adults, never by children.

Procedure:

Place a small portion of the suspected allergen in the sample holder and hold it in your palm, touching the jar with the fingertips of the same hand for 15 to 30 minutes. If you are allergic to the item in the jar, you will begin to feel uneasy when holding the allergen, giving rise to various unpleasant allergic symptoms, or exaggerating the prior allergic symptoms. The intensity of symptoms experienced is directly related to the severity of the allergy.

When one holds an allergen, one or more of the symptoms from the following list may be experienced:

Abdominal discomforts
Anger
Asthma
Backaches
Begins to get hot or cold on various parts of the body
Blurry eyes
Brain fog
Butterfly sensation in the stomach
Chest pains
Cough
Cravings
Crying spells
Deafness or ringing in the ear
Dry mouth, nose or throat
Fatigue
Flatulence
Frequency of urination
Headaches
Heaviness in the head
Heaviness in the chest
Heavy sensation in the body
Hives
Hyperactivity
Insomnia
Irregular heart beats (fast or slow)
Irritable
Itching in the nose, eyes, cheeks and ears
Knee or other joint pains
Light-headedness
Migraine headaches

Mucus in the throat
Nausea
Nervousness
Nose bleeds
Pin prick sensation
Pins and needles on the palms or soles
Poor attention span
Poor bowel control
Poor vision
Rashes
Redness on the cheeks and ears
Restlessness
Runny nose or blocked nostrils
Shortness of breath
Sinus troubles
Sneezing attacks
Sudden appearance of canker sores
Sudden eruption of acne or pimples on the face or body
Suddenly becomes silent
Suddenly becomes talkative
Unexplained pain anywhere in the body
Watering eyes
Weakness of any part of the limbs

Since the allergen is inside the sample-holder when such uncomfortable sensations are felt, the allergen can be put away immediately and the person can wash his/her hands to remove the energy of the allergen from the fingertips. This should stop the reaction immediately. In this way, you can determine allergens and the degree of allergy easily without putting yourself in danger.

NAET Testing Procedure #2

Testing and isolating a particular blockage can be done in many ways. One method, described below, is fairly easy to understand and, with some practice, can be mastered by anyone.

Subject and tester should wash their hands with soap and water before beginning the test, to remove any adverse energy from the fingertips.

Step 1: Balance the subject and find an indicator muscle. Refer to Chapter 6 to learn more about balancing and MRT.

Step 2: Patient lies down on his/her back with suspected allergen (e.g., an apple or item in sample-holder) in his/her resting palm. Use a surrogate when needed to test a child.

Step 3: Tester touches the points in diagram 8-1 one at a time, and tests the Pre-Determined Muscle (PDM) and compares the strength of the PDM in the absence and presence of the allergen. For example, touch point -1 in Figure 8-1 with the fingertips of one hand and with the other hand test the indicator muscle (while the patient is still holding the allergen in one hand). If the test muscle goes weak, it indicates the meridian, or the energy pathways connected to that particular point, has an energy disturbance.

Point -1 relates to the lung meridian. Obstruction in the energy flow anywhere in the lung meridian can make this point go weak. Table 8-1 is the description of the points in Figure 8-1. Test all other

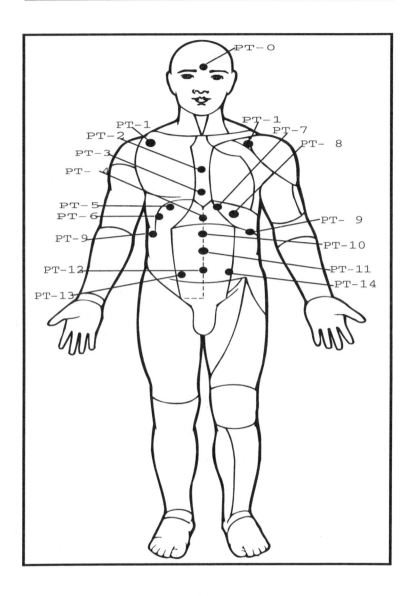

FIGURE 8-1
ACU THERAPY POINTS

Point Name	Related Meridian	Related organ
Pt - 0	Brain Test Pt	Brain
Pt -1	LU test pt	Lung
Pt - 2	P-HT (physical heart)	Pericardium
Pt - 3	HT test pt	Heart
Pt - 4	ST test pt	Stomach
Pt - 5	Liv test pt	Liver
Pt - 6	GB test pt	Gall bladder
Pt - 7	SP test pt	Spleen
Pt -8	Pan test pt	Pancreas
Pt - 9	Kid pt	Kidney
Pt - 10	SI ttest pt	Small intestine
Pt - 11	TW test point	Triple warmer
Pt - 12	Ut/Pr test pt	Uterus/prostate
Pt-13	Bl test pt	Bladder
Pt-14	LI test pt	Colon

TABLE 8-1
ACU THERAPY

points using this technique. Write down all the weak points. For point-meridian relationships, refer to Table 8-1. Using this technique, you can trace all weak meridians.

1. NAET Self-Help #1

Acu Therapy

Acu therapy can be used to restore the energy flow in the energy meridians by removing blockages.

Step 1: The first step for Acu therapy is to find the organ-associated test-point that is weak. Find the related organ test point in table 8-1, and in figure 8-1, then do MRT to locate the weak point.

Step 2: Apply slight finger pressure with the pad of your index finger on the weak point. Hold 60 seconds. Then move on to the next point following the numerical order. If you don't have weakness in any point, you can still use this technique to balance the body to improve the immune system. But if there is a weak organ point, make that a starting point to perform the energy balancing. For example, if the energy is blocked in the heart meridian, make the heart test point (point-3) the first point to begin the acu therapy, then the next will be points-4, 5, 6, 7, etc. If the liver is blocked, use the liver point (point-5) as the first point in the sequence of energy balancing. (If you do not know how to find the blocked point, start from point-1 and follow the order until you reach point-14, then massage the point-1 once again.)

Step 3: Hold 60 seconds at each point and go through all

14 points in the order given in figure 8-1 and finish the therapy at point-1 (beginning point). The starting point is treated twice. So, hold 60 seconds at the starting point before stopping the treatment.

Some patients can experience physical or emotional pain or an emotional release during these balancing sessions. If the patient has an emotional blockage, it needs to be isolated and balanced. Some patients can get tingling pains, sharp pains, pulsation, excessive perspiration, etc., during the energy balancing session. In such instances, please go through another cycle of treatment. This will often correct the problem. Some commonly used acupuncture points, and their uses to help in emergency situations are given below, with resuscitation point locations in Figure 8-5. Massage each of these points gently with the finger pads for one minute or until the problem in solved.

If you would like to learn more about acupuncture/acupressure points or about meridians, please refer to the suggested textbooks in the bibliography. Chapter 10 in my book "Say Good-bye to Illness," may also help.

Acu therapy can also help to keep your symptoms under control in these following situations:

Acute allergic reactions

Backache

Depression

Fatigue

Headache

Hyperactivity

Insomnia

Mood swings

Pain disorders

PMS (premenstrual symptoms)

Commonly seen children's disorders

It is a good idea to balance your body by applying Acu therapy or massaging the points clockwise, one minute on each points daily, twice a day. If you are very weak or sick, someone else can help to balance your points until you are strong enough to do so yourself.

You may also want to balance your points once or twice-a-day while you are going through NAET treatments with a practitioner. This will help you finish the treatments easier without having to repeat multiple times for the same allergen.

You don't have to be sick to benefit from balancing the body. You can use this balancing technique with or without NAET treatments. Using these points you can never overbalance the body or overtreat the meridians. One can never be too healthy. If you are already healthy, you can maintain your health by doing acu therapy regularly. If you are sick, have allergies, or are unhealthy for whatever reasons, by treating these points regularly, you will feel better.

This technique can also be used to balance the body not only in the morning or night, but any time you feel out of balance. How do you know if you are out of balance? If you are a healthy person, if your energy gets slightly out of balance you may not feel sick but may not feel quite right. You may feel tired, or sleepy in the afternoon, or not having the right motivation to do your work, etc., but you cannot find a definite reason for such "out of sorts" feeling. Some minor energy disturbance in the meridians may be the cause. If you can immediately balance the body using these points, you will clear the energy blockage and feel normal in minutes.

Acute Care

If a person is having an acute health problem (e.g. shortness of breath, abdominal pain, etc.), you can use acu therapy points to help bring the problem under control. Using the same method described above, massage these points or emergency points often until the problem is resolved or until help arrives.

Children can get sick very easily. You may balance your child using self-help #2. Allergy may be the cause for the child's sickness. The usual culprits include: food, drinks, clothes, toy, etc.

Find the allergen causing the immediate problem (asthma, sinus congestion, shortness of breath, fever, seizures, etc.) by testing with MRT, using the information from Chapter 6. If you are able to trace the causative allergen, place the substance in a sample-holder, and have the child touch the sample-holder as you balance using # 2 method.

NAET Self-Help #2

Back-Stroke Therapy

Look at the Figure 8-2. Have the child lie on a flat surface (perhaps on a table). Support the child or hold the child with one hand over his/her back (either clothed or unclothed). Keep the allergen in a sample-holder near the child, touching an exposed area of the body. Gently stroke from neck down (Level-1) to level of the waistline (level-2) as shown in Figure 8-2. 13 strokes are applied at one cycle. Repeat the cycles every ten minutes until the child feels better or until help arrives.

If you didn't call for emergency help, after the acute phase is over, and the child's condition is stabilized, make appointment with an NAET practitioner to get the NAET basic 15 to 25 groups treated. Clearing the NAET basic allergen groups will help prevent future similar attacks.

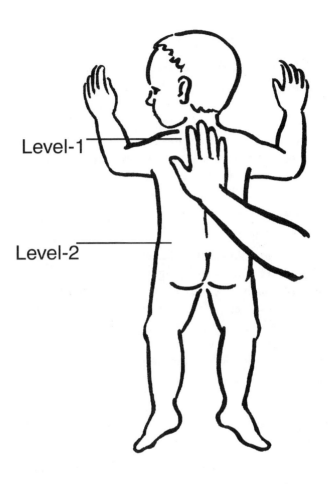

Figure 8-2
Back-Stroke Therapy

NAET Self-Help #3
Back-Stroke with Breathing

NAET Breathing Technique can be used to help with acute reactions

The person is asked to lie down on a flat surface, face down, holding the suspected allergen in his/her hand. This is the preferred position. If the person cannot lie down for any reason, he/she can sit down, crossing hands across the chest or touching the shoulders with opposite hands, back facing the helper.

Breathing technique is done in four steps (see procedure below for more specific instructions.)

1. Breathe in and hold while the helper applies one single back-stoke from level-1 to level-2 in figure 8-3.

2. Breathe out and hold while the helper applies another backstroke from level-1 to level-2 in figure 8-3.

3. Breathe fast (or pant) while the helper applies three quick backstrokes from level-1 to level-2 in figure 8-3.

4. Breathe normally while the helper applies two backstrokesfrom level-1 to level-2 in figure 8-3.

Balancing can begin with any of the first three steps. Fourth step is applied last.

Caution: Persons with known severe allergies should not hold the allergen sample in the hand when a friend or family member tries to balance this way. These patients with severe allergies should be treated by a qualified NAET Sp. only. People with these following disorders should not use breathing technique: shortness of breath, acute pulmonary disorders, acute cardiac disorders, very weak persons, very old persons, people with chronic illnesses.

Position: Patient can sit, stand or lie in prone position while doing this procedure. But the helper should make sure that the person is stable in whichever position he/she prefers. General balancing can be achieved if the backstroke therapy is applied without holding the allergen. If the sample is held by the patient while applying the backstrokes, the sensitivity of the allergen will be reduced.

Procedure:

Step 1: Ask the person to inhale and hold his/her breath while you apply the backstroke from level-1 to level-2. If the patient needs to stop to take a breath in between the backstrokes, stop for a few seconds halfway down the back, allow the person to take a quick breath out and in, then hold breath again, continue the treatment.

Step 2: Ask person to exhale and hold his/her breath while you apply backstroke. Again give a break halfway down the back if you need to.

Step 3: Ask the patient to breathe fast (at the rate of about 30 breaths per minute) while you apply backstrokes.

Step 4: Ask the patient to breathe normally while you apply backstroke.

Reasons for this specific pattern of breathing while applying backstrokes are as follows:

When you breathe-in, oxygenated, vibrant energy flows through each cell in the body. The allergen is introduced into the body in the presence of good, healthy energy.

When you breathe-out, deoxygenated, unhealthy, energy flows through each cell in the body. The allergen is introduced into the body in the presence of a toxic condition.

Breathing fast is mimicking the stressful condition of the body and when the body is made aware of the presence of the allergen in a stressful condition, the body will learn to handle the presence of the allergen in a stressful situation in the future.

Balancing the body with regular breathing is done to make the body aware of the presence of the allergen in a normal, relaxed, condition. After balancing the body with the allergen in these four conditions, a person's body will be able to face the allergen in all phases of life without adverse effects in the future.

Following this 4-step procedure, ask the person to lie in supine position, redo the MRT to verify the status of the previously recorded weak organs. If the organs remain weak, redo steps 1 through 4 until the organs test strong by MRT.

If the MRT is strong, balance the acu therapy points starting from point-1, go through all 14 points and end at point-1. This will balance the whole body including front and back part of the meridians.

Treating Viral Attack or "Flu"

If a child develops sudden "flu" or "viral attack," collect a sample of the saliva in a sample-holder and balance the child using back-stokes as described above. If you were able to do MRT and detect the causative allergen responsible for the sickness, (ear infection, fever or such illness), collect the allergen in a sample-holder and have the child hold the sample. Balance the child using self-help #2, every 10 minutes until he/she gets better or until the help arrives.

Childhood vomiting, diarrhea, ear infection, colds and flu's, fever, sinus troubles, hives, cough, abdominal pains after meals, etc., are commonly seen. Test everything child ate or drank during the previous 25 hours. Put samples in a sample-holder. Have the child lie down on a flat area (table) as in the Figure 8-2, hold the sample touching the child's body while you balance him/her using the backstrokes. If the exact causative allergen is not available, collect a

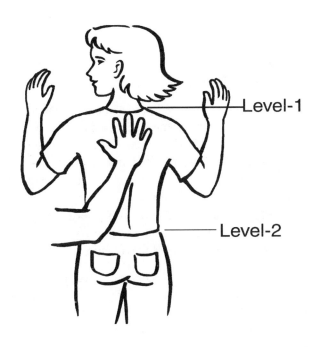

FIGURE 8-3
BACK-STROKE WITH BREATHING

small sample of the child's discharge in a sample-holder (example: sample of vomitus, nasal discharge, stool, sweat, etc.) then balance the child's energy.

Acute Allergic Reactions

If you get an acute reaction to some food you ate in a restaurant or at home, or by coming in contact with an allergen, if you know the causative allergen, you may hold it in a sample-holder to balance your body using any of the three methods described above. You may repeat the balancing treatments ten minutes apart until you feel better. By treating this way, you may not clear the allergy permanently but you could control your allergic symptoms temporarily. When you stabilize your condition you should go to the appropriate medical practitioner for evaluation.

As you have seen from the above description of energy balancing procedures, you can achieve good results by balancing acu-points on the front or back of the body. They both give similar results if done properly. When you balance your energy on your own, front acu-points are convenient to work with. But if you are helping someone else to balance his/her energy you may use the backstroke- technique, which can be applied to children as well as adults.

Severe Allergic Reactions and/or Anaphylaxis

<u>Rules for Treating Anaphylactic Patients in the Office</u>

• Please do not try self-help treatments at home on patients with a history of anaphylaxis. Find a qualified NAET specialist to get the following treatments.

• The practitioner should complete at least fifteen Basic NAET allergen groups before attempting to treat for any known anaphylactic items. These patients should not try to self-treat. Have the treatments done by a qualified NAET specialist. You can never be too careful when it comes to your health. You can completely eliminate the anaphylactic reactions through NAET if done carefully and properly. The following golden rules should be observed:

• Always test and treat the person through a surrogate only.

• Do not let the person touch the sample directly.

• Have the sample in a sample-holder, and let the surrogate hold it in the far hand, away from the person while testing and treating.

• While checking for weak areas, the patient remains away from the hand of the surrogate in which the sample is held.

• After the treatment, the patient should not hold the sample for the usual 20 minutes.

• Ask the patient to massage on the general balancing points (Figure 8-4) every 2 hours during the 25 hours following the treatment.

- Follow the rest of the instructions for a regular NAET treatment. Your practitioner will explain the rest to you at the time of the treatment.

On the next visit, check the item thoroughly for the organs, levels, and possible combinations and, if needed, the NAET specialist should treat for all the necessary combinations as many times as needed until the NAET specialist is satisfied with the result. In some extremely severe cases, it has taken 10-15 treatments (one treatment per day) to eliminate an allergy to an item (example-peanut) that has caused anaphylactic reactions in the past.

Some of the items treated successfully with NAET and with no further reactions are: penicillin, aspirin, mushroom, shellfish, peanuts, milk, egg, iodine, hair dye, perfume, formaldehyde, bee stings, and latex.

After completion of the NAET on the anaphylactic item, if the practitioner cannot find any more combinations, have the patient hold the item in a sample-holder and sit in the practitioner's office for half-an-hour every day for a week. After that, let the patient hold the item in his/her hand without the holder every day for half-an-hour to an hour for a week. If the patient does not show any more adverse symptoms when contacted, then on the next visit, he/she can put a small portion of it in the mouth and wait for a few minutes, then spit it out and rinse the mouth with clear water. Do this everyday for a week. If the patient did not have any reaction during this observation period, if the patient wants to consume the item, he/she will be able to do so now.

Even after clearing the allergy satisfactorily, every new batch of the item should be checked for possible allergy and treated if necessary. One can never be too careful when it comes to health, especially regarding severe allergy.

In cases of peanut or peanut butter allergies, you don't have to make the child eat a peanut butter sandwich every day, but the

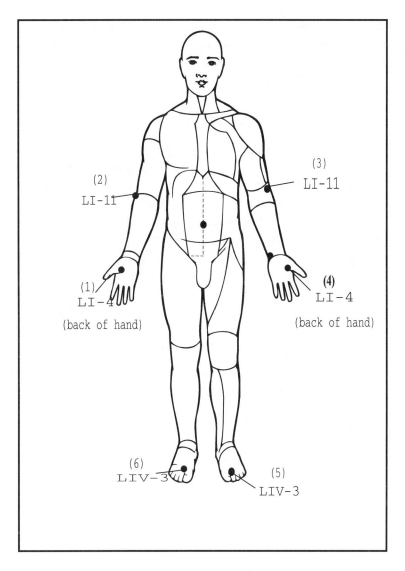

FIGURE 8-4

GENERAL BALANCING POINTS

treatment is mainly for preventing anaphylaxis and other unpleasant reactions when the child is among other people in the neighborhood who are eating peanut products.

General Balancing Technique

Look at the Figure 8-4. Massage these points gently for a minute each, clockwise, in circular motion with your fingerpads starting from point-1, go through pt-2, pt-3, pt-4, pt-5,pt-6, and finish up the massage at point-1. A point stimulator may be used in place of finger massage. Massaging these points can improve the nerve energy circulation in the meridians. Treating these points will increase your overall energy. After each NAET treatment, these points should be massaged or needled to balance the body to help the NAET treatment last long.

The Oriental Medicine CPR Point

The CPR (Cardiopulmonary rescscitation) point of Oriental Medicine is the Governing Vessel-26.

Location: Below the nose, a little above the midpoint of the philtrum.

Indication: Fainting, sudden loss of consciousness, cardiac arrhythmia, heart attack, stroke, sudden loss of energy, hypoglycemia, heatstroke, sudden pain in the lower back, general lower backache, breathing problem due to allergic reactions, mental confusion, mental irritability, anger, uncontrollable rage, exercise-induced anaphylaxis, anaphylactic reactions to allergens, and sudden breathing problem due to any cause.

Procedure: Massage or stimulate the point for 30 seconds to a minute at the beginning of the problem.

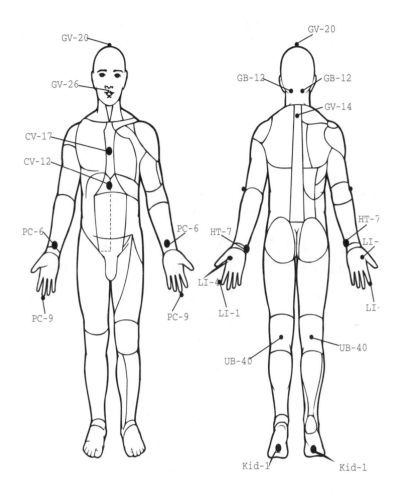

Figure 8-5
Resuscitation Points

• If you are treating yourself to wake up from sleeping while driving, or to recover from sudden loss of energy, etc., massage gently on this point. For example: While you are driving, if you feel sudden loss of energy or sensation of fainting, immediately massage this point. Your energy will begin to circulate faster and you will prevent a fainting episode.

• If you are reviving an unconscious victim who passed out in front of you, you may massage the point vigorously to inflict slight pain so that the person will wake up immediately. Vigorous massage is used only to wake up the fainted person or the person who became unresponsive in front of you.

Points to Help With Medical Emergencies

1. Fainting: GV-20, GV-26, GB-12, LI-1, PC-9, Kid-1

2. Nausea: CV-12, PC-6, Ht-7

3. Backache: GV-26, UB-40

4. Fatigue: CV-6, LI-1, CV-17, Liv-3

5. Fever: LI-11, GV-14

Stimulate these points by massaging them clockwise one at a time (from right to left on the patient's body) as you need them to control acute symptoms. Patients will usually respond within 30 seconds to one minute of stimulating these points. If someone is slow to respond, it is OK to massage for three to five minutes. But please stop and evaluate the condition of the patient every 30 seconds.

Do not hesitate to call for emergency help (911), if you ever need it.

For more information on revival points, refer to Chapter 3, pages 570 to 573, in "Acupuncture: A Comprehensive Text," by Shanghai College of Traditional Medicine, Eastland Press, 1981, or refer to my book, "Living Pain Free with Acupressure," 1997, available at various bookstores and at our website **naet.com**

A Word to the Allergic Patient

I have attempted to discuss most of the various types of allergic manifestations, the more common types of allergic reactions, and the prevalent Western and Oriental diagnostic and treatment methods of allergies. I have presented sufficient information on NAET to free you from your immediate allergic reactions to the allergens you come in contact with in your everyday life. I have also explained in detail how to test and find your allergies on your own—with the most reliable and least expensive method of allergy testing. If studied carefully, this information should help allergic patients control allergic reactions and prevent unexpected and unfortunate incidences.

It is hoped that you will spend some time carefully rereading every page related to testing and balancing techniques. Mild reactions can be treated using these techniques. However, they do not replace the need for visiting your allergist or an NAET practitioner. After you overcome an immediate emergency situation using the methods herein, please make an appointment with your doctor to manage the rest of your problems. Please do not take the responsibility on yourself to continue to treat your allergies without the help of a trained practitioner. Please do not forget that these medical practitioners have sacrificed thousands of hours in medical schools to learn how to help you and to provide you with a comfortable journey towards wellness. You cannot expect to replace their knowledge with this book.

I hope you will take enough time to understand the material presented herein, to learn about NTT and MRT, to detect your allergies and to make use of the balancing techniques. In addition, it is important for you to know and understand the emergency measures that will help you in any emergency situations. NAET specialists are available at various locations throughout the country and elsewhere in world. I cannot emphasize enough the importance of full and complete cooperation between you and your practitioner. It is only by such cooperation that you can obtain the best results.

It is not sufficient for the patient to only receive regular treatments, although this is vitally important. He/she must also follow the other instructions if he/she hopes to attain the maximum result in a minimum time. My book, The NAET Guide Book, should be read by all NAET patients. This book gives step-by-step instructions to follow during the 24 hours after NAET. Most NAET allergy treatments require repeated office visits in the beginning. Once all the known allergens are eliminated, patients are trained to find their own allergens and self-treat the minor ones as and when they appear. They have to see the doctor only if a reaction to an item that bothers them can't be eliminated using the self-help methods, or for annual follow-ups. All allergens cannot be eliminated in one or two office visits. In some severe cases, it may take as many as three visits a week for one or two years or more to achieve a condition close to normalcy. This is contingent on the patient's immune system response.

Allergic patients should keep this time span in mind when they approach any NAET specialist. If treatment is discontinued before completion of all the necessary basic treatments, the results will be unsatisfactory and allergic symptoms are very likely to recur. This may tend to make the patient feel that the treatment is useless. For this reason, it is better not even to start treatment than to start and discontinue too soon, or to start and then cooperate halfheartedly. The NAET practitioner will discharge patients just as soon as it is safe to do so.

How can patients cooperate and help the doctor achieve maximum results in minimum time? After each treatment, patients are advised to stay away from the treated item for 25 hours. There are

12 energy meridians. It takes two hours for an energy molecule to pass through one meridian. To circulate through 12 meridians takes 24 hours. This means that the patient should not even come close to the object during that time, as its electromagnetic field can interfere with the patient's own field and negate the treatment.

Patients are advised to maintain a food diary. If the patient violently reacts to something while going through the treatment program, the offender can easily be traced and treated, preventing further pain. Patients are placed on a strict diet of non-allergic items after completion of the first three basic treatments. This helps the body to detoxify the accumulated toxins prior to the treatments. This also helps maintain good health without having to face possible allergic items. It also speeds up the treatment process while reducing interference.

Statistics show that from 80 to 90 percent of allergic patients who receive proper NAET treatments, and cooperate with the doctor, are either entirely relieved of any allergy-related problems or are satisfactorily improved. NAET treatment can provide satisfying results if done properly.

CHAPTER 9

Doctors' Testimonials

As a neurologist, I have seen many diseases as a direct result of allergies. I knew of no other better way of locating allergies successfully, which is natural, safe, non-invasive and drug-free. It treats most common and uncommon allergies in the most efficient way in few minutes.

Ravinder Singh, M.D.
Singh Neurology Medical Group
Beverly Hills, California
(310) 278-4171
email: singh@singhneurology.com

"Allergy ELIMINATION?!? Is it possible?" I asked when I first heard about Dr. Devi and NAET. "Absolutely!" is the answer to that question I later discovered after meeting Devi and learning her amazingly simple, most effective technique. Bar none, no other allergy treatment in my practice has been as effective as NAET. Dr. Devi is truly a medical pioneer, and she has my deepest respect, both personally and professionally. TELL EVERYONE YOU KNOW about the best-kept secret in the world of allergy diagnosis and therapy: NAET.

NAET Sp: Ann McCombs, D.O.
Medical Director
Center for Optimum Health
Seattle, Washington
(425) 576- 0951

NAET is truly awesome. You will want to pass this book on to others and spread the word about this amazing technique. Anyone who has wrestled with a rotation diet or tried to eliminate wheat, sugar, and dairy from a small child's diet knows what a struggle that can be. But with the NAET process all of this becomes unnecessary. An allergen can be eliminated within 25 hours of treatment! No more having to avoid the food. By finding an NAET practitioner in your area, and following through with the treatments, you and your child can get a new lease on life and tackle new horizons.

NAET Sp: Sandra C. Denton, M.D.
Clinical Ecologist
Alaska Alternative Medical Center
Anchorage, Alaska
(907) 563-6200

NAET is a powerful and natural, interactive technique that engages the patients' participation in order to attain successful results. NAET offers solutions to some of the most difficult, odd and troublesome health issues that traditional medicine often fails to address. NAET provides resolution to those patients who have slipped through the cracks of modern medicine. For those who have suffered pain and restriction in their lives and functioning, NAET delivers the freedom of a more normal life and life style. NAET is the most revolutionary natural health technique of the end of the last century, and millions of now healthy patients around the world owe a great debt to Dr. Devi Nambudripad for her brilliant intellect and creative insights.

Rahmie Valentine, O.M.D., L.Ac., Ph.D.
(323) 931-7387
Rahmie@aol.com

Much of my practice involves working with children and adults with ADD, ADHD, OCD and learning disabilities. After treating them for allergies using NAET, I have witnessed tremendous results. The children look forward to the treatments and the parents have restored hope after years of frustration.

NAET Sp: Carol Perkins, N.D.
Lexington, Kentucky
(859) 277-5255

Your accomplishment of the development of NAET is a great contribution to the science of energy medicine. Many of us are indebted to you for the introduction of energy medicine to us. Many thousands of patients have benefited. I have adapted the benefits of NAET to my practice of ophthalmology and have been able to see therapeutic results not available with traditional Western medicine. Congratulations and thanks for your accomplishments and sharing with us selflessly.

NAET Sp: Paul R. Honan, M.D.
Lebanon, Indiana
(765) 482-1954

The NAET eye mix treatment has had an amazing affect on one of my toddler patients on his "lazy" eye (strabismus) condition. After the eye mix treatment, his eye began to move toward center after being fixed in the inside corner of the eye. The eye has started to track objects and he has become much more interested in visually exploring his environment. NAET is Incredible!

NAET Sp: Marcia Costello, R.N., M. Ac., L.Ac.
Marlborough, Massachusetts
(508) 786-0788

I have been practicing anesthesiology and pain management for the past 12 years. My four-year-old son has been freed from being labeled "autistic" through NAET. Dr. Nambudripad's NAET has literally restored our family's physical and emotional health. I have witnessed disabled patients who had failed many other modalities respond wonderfully with NAET. No doubt that I had failed to find the cause of so many illnesses since I was too busy writing prescriptions to treat symptoms! NAET should be practiced by all the health-care professionals who sincerely care about the patients.

NAET Sp: Lisa Camerino, M.D.
Anesthesiologist, NAET Practitioner
Portland, Oregon
(503) 805-2112

One morning, I woke up with a terrible sinus headache. I was about ready to take some Ibuprofen so that I could function at work. But then it occurred to me that I could use MRT to find out what was causing the pain. It turned out to be some Thai chicken I had the day before. I had some leftover in the fridge. After an NAET treatment for Thai chicken, the pain dissipated by 50% within 15 minutes. And within one hour the headache was gone completely.

NAET Sp: Ann M. Auburn, D.O.
Board Certified Family Practice
and Osteopathic Manipulative Medicine
3700-52nd St. S.E., Grand Rapids, Michigan 49316
(616) 656-3700

I have been especially impressed with the use of NAET in eliminating food allergies. We have seen people who had to avoid certain foods for years such as chocolates, nuts, tomatoes, etc. who can eat these items comfortably after being cleared on them with NAET. This is especially remarkable when we consider that conventional allergists recommend that persons with food allergies should avoid the allergic substances for the remainder of their lives.

One young man had been afflicted with severe reactions to crab meat for years, and would have to eat non-seafood items when his family went to a traditional all-you-can-eat crab broil around Thanksgiving each year. After he received NAET clearing for seafood, I saw him at a family gathering about a month later and asked how his NAET treatment was holding up. He said, "I've been making up for ten years of lost time." I like to think of NAET as the ultimate technique for dealing with food allergies.

NAET Sp: Robert Prince, M.D.
Charlotte, North Carolina

I had a very nice lady named Nadia come to the office with red, swollen, canker sores that were very painful and would pop up in her mouth every time she had a food or drink that was acidic. She had this since childhood. After the basic NAET treatments, they cleared up and she can eat anything and even use vinegar with no problems.

NAET Sp: James Aylor, D.C., N.D.
816 Camarillo Springs Road, Suite A
Camarillo, California 93010
(805) 987-1800

In February, 2002, a patient at our center was being seen for vomiting which was occurring daily since 9/11. She worked downtown and saw the second plane hit. She had already been seen by a gastroenterologist who found no cause for her vomiting. I was called by the practitioner seeing her to treat her for the emotional allergy to what she witnessed. Following the treatment, the vomiting stopped.

NAET Sp: Geri Brewster R.D., M.P.H., C.D.N.
The Atkins Center for Complimentary Medicine
24 West 57th Street, 7th Floor, Manhattan, NY 10019
(212) 977-9870

I went to my dentist for removal of an old silver amalgam filling. Immediately after the removal of old amalgam and replacement with a new porcelain composite, I felt the inside of my cheek inflamed, with a layer of tissue peeled off. I thought that I had bitten my cheek. After two days it was still the same. A friend mentioned that he had a similar allergic reaction a couple of years ago, when he had the same procedure. I was reminded to check for my own allergy. Sure enough, I found myself very allergic to amalgam, especially to mercury. I immediately treated myself for mercury and amalgam using NAET. After 26 hours of the treatment, I had no discomfort in my cheek. The lesion healed nicely. NAET again brought me back to health. Thank You!

> NAET Sp: Roger Valentine, D.V.M.
> Pet Allergy Center
> Santa Monica, California

I thought you might rejoice sharing this boy's happiness. Kevin was unable to eat eggs. When he ate any products with eggs in them, his mouth turned into fire, his throat swelled, and he had to be rushed to the hospital ER or given an epipen injection. He was unable to enjoy birthday cakes and other delights made with eggs for four of his seven years. After his first NAET clearing for eggs, he was able to have a small egg product. After clearing many combinations associated with eggs, including mayonnaise, cake frosting, stomach acid, grains and finally soybean oil and lecithin, Kevin is now able to eat any egg products — as much as he wants — without any reaction whatsoever. He's one very happy child, thanks to NAET!"

> NAET Sp: Gary Erkfritz, D.C.
> Thousand Oaks, California
> (805) 371-8082

I am so thrilled to have found NAET. NAET is the answer to my longtime quest for additional tools to rewire energy blockage and to correct energy unbalance, besides acupuncture and Chinese herbs. According to Chinese Medicine, all illnesses are caused by energy blockage and unbalance. We humans are energy beings. Energy flows within us as real as blood circulates within blood vessels. Balanced energy flow is the key for our well-being. Unfortunately, in our daily life, emotions, foods, and environmental hazards are causing energy blockage and unbalance consistently. That's why even thousands of years ago Chinese doctors stated that emotions, foods, and environmental hazards are the only cause of illness. Thanks to Dr. Nambudripad, with her NAET, removing specific blockage becomes such an easy task. I have witnessed amazing healing with many of my patients through NAET treatment. Thanks to Dr. Nambudripad from me and from all my NAET patients.

NAET Sp: Iris Chen, A.P., M.D., Ph.D.

Incredible Herbs and Acupuncture
6245 North Federal Highway, #202
Fort Lauderdale, Florida 33308
(954) 771-1007

I have known Devi for twenty years, since our mutual days in chiropractic and acupuncture schools. She has made a lasting impression on the lives of thousands of people, and I am proud to be associated with her. I will continue to help as many people as I can with this simple, direct and effective system that she developed. Dr. Devi is changing lives and making some lives worth living; what can be more rewarding and worthwhile than that?

I have been using NAET in my practice for the past 5-6 years. At first, I was somewhat skeptical: after all, how could such a simple system have such dramatic results when other, more traditional and accepted treatments have been unsuccessful. However, it is impossible to deny the efficacy of something that has allowed a

34-year-old, severely asthmatic man to play with cats for the first time in his life. Or allow a five-year-old boy to eat like a normal child rather than to break out in hives when most foods touch his lips. Even more dramatically, NAET helped a six-year-old 'autistic' girl who was unable to speak or play or join others her own age in normal children's activities. I am convinced and so are my patients.

NAET Sp: Susan Meisinger D.C., L.Ac.
Woodland Hills, California
(818) 883-1242

I was treated with NAET during my first pregnancy, with amazing results. My chronic rhinitis of five years was resolved in four treatments. I decided to learn this technique to be able to provide myself, my family and my patients with a comprehensive treatment for allergies. Within a few days of NAET Basic Seminar I was able to treat myself for an acute shoulder pain and my son for a sudden cough, both resulted from eating allergic foods. NAET is a revolutionary means of evaluating and treating allergies painlessly, without risk. This is definitely going to be THE Medicine of the FUTURE!

NAET Sp: Gracie Lyons, M.D.
Board Certified OB GYN
Phoenix, Arizona
JAMES GBH@aol.com

This simple, yet powerful, technique saved my life. I now enjoy LIVING! My family, friends and patients experience a wellness that they had not known, some of them for years. The energy of the body and mind flowing freely is the true expression of LIFE... God Bless You, Dr. Devi!

NAET Sp: Barbara Cesmat, DCH, Ph.D.
Woodland Hills, California

We had a fantastic change in a patient using NAET and wanted to let you know. She is a 50-year-old woman who is a RN and runs a medical office near us. She had severe Diabetes for two years and has been on two oral hypoglycemics and a very strict low carbohydrate diet. She got her NAET basic ten and then we determined the combination treatment with sugar. After completing the combination treatment with sugar, insulin, pancreas, and stomach acid she woke up the next morning with a blood sugar of 80. She has not had any diabetic medicine for over two weeks and her sugars have remained normal! She has even started eating bread and potatoes, and the sugar level remains within normal range.

NAET Sp: David Minkoff, M.D.
Clearwater, Florida
(727) 466-6789

My first autistic patient was a 29-year-old autistic adult. When he began treatment with me, he was unable to communicate with anyone about his needs. He was incontinent and was on diapers. He behaved like a two-year-old. When he finished the first five NAET basic treatments, he was able to communicate with his parents asking for his favorite food - ice cream. When he finished the mineral mix treatment, he stopped his bladder incontinence. By the time he completed his basic fifteen treatments, he was on his way to recovery. Step-by-step, little by little, I watched how NAET transformed a violent, frustrated, autistic child into a passive, focused, manageable state. Ever since I have seen many autistic patients go through similar processes. When children get the NAET treatments at a younger age the result is phenomenal. NAET is a simple technique but it is so powerful beyond imagination!

NAET Sp: Mala Moosad, R.N., L.Ac., N.D.
Buena Park, California
(714) 523-8900

My patient had constantly recurring bladder infections for the past five years due to a prolapsed bladder. Acupuncture helped, but with NAET the infections have stopped!

NAET Sp: Pam Mills, L.Ac
4310 N.Troy
Chicago, Illinois 60618
(773) 588-2912

A co-worker of mine has had Raynaud's disease for over 20 years. I treated her for the basics, and when we finished the iron treatment, she noticed an immediate improvement in her hands and feet. After boosting her body with iron supplements, she no longer experiences any symptoms of Raynaud's at all. On top of this, after her salt mix treatment, her arthritis had improved almost 100%. NAET is amazing. Thank you Dr. Devi for discovering NAET.

NAET Sp: Tami Breichnge, R.N.
Mahtomedi, Minnesota

NAET is truly the medicine of the future. It is exciting to be using it in the present. The results and satisfaction are mind boggling. I can hardly believe it, even though I see the results over and over again, each and every day. The scope of the many health problems that NAET routinely helps continues to astound me, and amazes my patients. The only problem is there are not enough hours now to treat the many patients wanting treatment with this wonderful technique.

NAET Sp: Terry Power
BSc., Grad DC, M. ChiroSc, D. Ac.
Port Macquarie
NSW, Australia

NAET is a highly effective treatment for eliminating allergies in children. After the treatment, children are free to eat their favorite food without any adverse reaction. No needles, no pain!

NAET Sp: Peter Gao,
D.Ac, C.M.D., M.Sc.
Toronto, Ontario, Canada

One day my patient Dio called me. He was in a near hysterical state with fear. His doctor had just referred him to a neurologist and ordered an MRI exam for his brain. He told me he was to be evaluated for possible brain lesion and multiple sclerosis. His symptoms included restless leg syndrome and leg pain which kept him awake every night for six months. He had episodes of sudden weakness in his legs causing him to fall down while walking to the bathroom at night. Dio had allergies with nasal symptoms for many years. He was not helped by densensitization shots, sinus surgery or nasal surgery.

I asked him if he wanted to try NAET. After four NAET treatments and a couple of minor dietary changes, his symptoms diminished. He was free of pain, his leg muscle became strong, and he sleeps well again. His tremendous fear for his health has disappeared and he is in his old easy-going, smiling "Self" again. My patient Dio and I are so grateful to Dr. Devi and NAET. Thank You!

NAET Sp: Kathleen Sorensen, L.Ac, R.N.
West Palm Beach, Florida.
(561) 689-1480

NAET has given me even greater thrills in healing than chiropractic alone. Many patients are suffering a life of hell when they begin their therapy. Each allergy elimination brings them better health, and certainly more comfort. Never do you promote the therapy; it sells itself so naturally. Beautiful, holistic healing.

NAET Sp: Kate Willesee B.Sc., D.C.

Mosman, NSW, Australia

Since I have started treating patients with NAET, the results have been phenomenal, greater than my wildest expectations. Children who had life threatening allergies (asthma) are now symptom-free. Young adults who were unable to go to university, school, or even walk down the street because they were hypersensitive to the environment, can now go to nightclubs without ill effect. My practice has expanded by at least 200% since treating patients with NAET. Thank you, Devi, for coming to Australia and imparting this wonderful technique which has enabled me to bring health to my patients.

NAET Sp: Maria Colosimo N.D.
Melbourne, Australia

One of my patients, a 48-year-old female, was diagnosed as having M.S. (Multiple Sclerosis) 20 years back. She had been treated in my office for the past four years with chiropractic and acupuncture with significant improvement in her quality of life. A blood allergy test was performed four years ago which showed severe allergy to garlic. She has avoided garlic since but still she will get a severe headache if she even walks into a room with garlic smell. After three NAET treatments (BBF, egg mix and calcium mix), she commented she feels better than she felt in twenty years. She had increased clarity of mind, increased overall energy, and no more headaches. She said, "I was living on aspirins all these years." On her last visit, she said she is ready for Garlic, which she was initially planning to skip due to fear. But now she is convinced that NAET works and she is no longer fearful to go through NAET treatments for any type of allergens. She hopes her 20-year- M.S. will be history very soon.

NAET Sp: Uma Mulnick, D.C.
201 Park St , McCall, Idaho 83638
(208) 634-8129, muln@etcweb.net

My son, Evan, who, three years ago had an anaphylactic shock when he was stung by a bee, was stung again by a bee about two weeks ago. I have treated him with NAET for anaphylaxis to bee stings since the original sting. His reaction to the recent bee sting was a red wheel at the site of the sting. But he did not need the anaphylaxis treatment and he is doing fine.

Thank you, Dr. Devi, Mala, Mohan for teaching me this fabulous NAET treatment technique, so that I could cure my child from his severe anaphylactic reaction to bee stings, that is not treated successfully to full recovery by any other medical disciplines.

NAET Sp: Anthony DeSiena, D.C.
Eugene, Oregon 97401
(541) 686-BACK (2225)

I have treated many cases of Pollen allergies (Kafun Shou) and environmental allergies successfully with NAET. The following year, none of them had any problems with pollens in our heavy pollen season.

NAET Sp: Teruaki Nozawa, D.C.
2-4 Mitojima-honcho
Fuji-city, Shizuoka
Japan 416-0924

Dr. Devi's method has brought the understanding and approach to healing to a deeper level. It still puzzles me everyday how easily and thoroughly my patients are relieved of symptoms, layer after layer, and can enjoy a healthy life again — or, in some cases, experience it for the first time. There is no turning back now. Medicine can only progress from here.

NAET Sp: Frederique Nault, N.D.
Bali, Indonesia

A patient of mine was highly allergic to latex. She dreaded going to the dentist because after every dental appointment, her facial muscles would cramp and she would develop a rash around her mouth. I treated her for latex and after two treatments, she cleared the latex. Her next visit to her dentist was a success. She had no allergic reaction to the latex gloves!

Dr. Cade Caselman, D.C.,
Salina, Kansas (785) 867-1101

NAET has changed my life and practice. NAET is a profound and fascinating technique of correcting allergies, which is an underlying cause of most health problems and diseases.

NAET Sp: Sue Anderson, D.C.
Ann Arbor, MI
(734) 973-9692

I have been on the lookout for a technique which could deliver better results for my patients. With Dr. Devi and NAET, this has become a possibility. I believe a technique is only as good as the long-term results it produces. Even after a year of using NAET every day, I am still astounded by the results it is producing. For the first time in my chiropractic career I now feel, that by incorporating NAET into my practice, I can offer my patients totally holistic "WELLNESS" Care.

NAET Sp: Phil Barham, D.C.
Brisbane, Australia

Beginning NAET I soon learned I was actually allergic to almost everything in life. Pretty much the only thing I was not allergic to was my one-year-old daughter, and the results of the testing made sense of my experience of life. I knew I had a very strong body and yet I avoided lots of foods to avoid what I now know to be allergic symptoms. Mainly, my allergies had been showing up as brain fog and various emotional reactions, some of which I had just put down to how I was.

Even more powerful for me than the food and environmental treatments, has been emotional and interpersonal allergies and having them treated and cleared. My partner and I were both allergic to each other (recipe for a fiery relationship, to say the least) and clearing these has definitely been one of the biggest and most special allergies to have cleared. The results show there in our improved relating with each other. As a medical doctor, I have long had dreams of transforming the current medical health system, knowing through experience many of its limitations. So I am very excited about now passing on the benefits of NAET to others.

I particularly love NAET in that I have always felt that the real role of a doctor is to assist people in their own healing, helping the body do what it knows how to do, which is to operate in a state of health that is in harmony with all of life. NAET opens the door to this and the results, which touch every level of human experience, are very special. It is very special also to have NAET there as a tool to use with my one-year-old daughter, Leteitia. She developed a fairly severe bout of candida as a nappy rash, and it wasn't responding well to the anti-fungal lotion. I treated her for the candida vial using NAET and her rash went away that night. She has been free of it since. NAET is so simple and in my experience children, in particular, respond very quickly.

NAET Sp: Marcia Smart M.B.B.S.
Melbourne, Australia

Devi Nambudripad has generously shared her fascinating discovery of eliminating allergies so that we may all benefit from a healthy, allergy-free life. This is an important book that will bring blessed relief to many people.

NAET Sp: Debbie Carroll, R.N., D.Ac.,
New Brunswick, Canada

In our experience as one of the major research and treatment centers for Chronic Fatigue Syndrome and fibromyalgia, we have proven that effective treatment is now available for those with fatigue, pain, "brain fog" and insomnia. Our placebo-controlled study shows that 91% of patients improve (average improvement in quality of life of 90%) when one aggressively looks for and treats the underlying causes. By combining NAET with natural metabolic therapies, not only do over 90% of patients improve, a large percent no longer qualify as having CFS or fibromyalgia by the end of treatment! Most CFS/Fibromyalgia patients have multiple sensitivities to food, medications and environmental exposures which can both cause their symptoms and limit the effectiveness of treatment. NAET can be dramatically beneficial in treating the sensitivities, allowing patients to tolerate treatment, while testing for and clearing multiple sensitivities and infections. In fact, we consider NAET developed by Dr. Nambudripad to be where the medicine of the future is going. Because of this, we look forward to donating part of the royalties for the products we've developed (Daily Energy Enfusion powder which replaces 25 supplement tablets a day with a good tasting drink and Revitalising Sleep Formula for sleep-available at health food stores, NAET practitioners, or from www.endfatigue.com-100% of our royalties go to charity) to the NAET research fund as I believe NAET is one of the most powerful, safe and effective new treatments available. In fact , by combining NAET and metabolic therapies you can get vibrant and healthy again!

Many find NAET to be a miracle in their lives!

Best wishes,

NAET Sp: Laurie Teitelbaum
NAET Sp: Jacob Teitelbaum M.D.
Directors of the Annapolis Research Center for
Effective CFS/Fibromyalgia Therapies.
Author of the best selling book *From Fatigued to Fantastic!*"
and *"Three Steps to Happiness! Healing Through Joy"*

(410) 573-5389
www.EndFatigue.com

My patient had a severe case of eczema with oozing pus along his inner arms and thighs, which also caused extreme itching and considerable pain. He experienced depression and brain fog. Before coming to see me, he tried different treatment modalities but his condition was getting worse. After 12 NAET treatments, his eczema has decreased by 85%, oozing is stopped completely, with occasional itching. His mood is much more positive and his mind is clear.

I am grateful for Dr. Devi's generosity in sharing this knowledge with so many practitioners, who in turn use the treatment protocol to improve the well-being of even more people. From my personal contact with De, Devi, I experienced her as a genuinely sincere and caring person. Thank you Dr. Devi!

NAET Sp: Ming Chiu, L.Ac., D.Hom, CNC, MTOM, NCCA
2818 Santa Monica Blvd.
Santa Monica, California 90404
(310) 739-3166 / email: mingchiulac@aol.com

Dr. "Devi" has developed an amazingly effective treatment technique which continues to bring relief to thousands of patients. That is why I chose to become involved with NARF, the foundation that is dedicated to clinical trials and research in allergy elimination using NAET.

Based on our preliminary clinical research results, as well as the numerous case studies presented from around the world, NAET works on many levels to improve the lives of those it touches. I foresee widespread acceptance of NAET as we continue to obtain excellent results in our clinical research studies.

NAET Sp: Robert Cohen, M.D.
Research Director
NARF (Nambudripad's Allergy Research Foundation)
6714 Beach Blvd.Buena Park, California

I once had two children with multiple food and environmental allergies. One of these precious children was also classified PDD/mild autism. Although many alternative treatments helped him, his allergies would cause regression and our lifestyle was becoming almost unbearable. When I learned about NAET I was so happy I cried. Needless to say I did what I had to, got trained, and began to treat both of my children. Now I have two healthy children with no allergies! The child that was once classified is now mainstreamed and on the honor roll! I now treat many children with ADD, ADHD, and Autism and see remarkable results. Thank you Devi, you have made such a difference in so many lives. Thank you for saving so many children and their families too!

Maribeth Mydlowski, D.C.
Hamilton Township, NJ

CHAPTER 10

Case Studies

Case Study: Fear Caused Ulcer in the Esophagus

Four-year-old Steven suffered from severe esophageal ulcers and inflammation for 11 months. He was evaluated, examined and treated by a few specialists in the nearby university hospitals. The child's esophageal ulcers remained a mystery to them. Since the whole esophagus was ulcerated, even surgery was out of question. The child couldn't eat or drink anything due to the severe pain he experienced from the throat down. He had a five-month-old brother on breast milk. His mother began breast feeding Steven again since he didn't hurt much on breast milk. Steven began losing weight. His worried parents frantically began looking for help everywhere. They found NAET through the website and brought Steven to our office for treatment.

While he was getting treated for a sugar allergy, he had to be treated for fear in order to clear the sugar treatment. His fear was traced back to the September 11, 2001, WTC incident. Why should a California-born, three-year- old be so fearful about the 9/11, causing such a strange health problem? It puzzled us. So we asked the mother to think back and tell us everything that happened on that day.

Then his mother remembered: His father who travels frequently for his business was flying from New York to Los Angeles at the time the airplanes attacked the WTC. His mother and grandmothers were terrified, not getting any communication from his father for hours. The child saw the panic in the family and became very fearful, and began throwing up right away, one of the reactions of fear and nervousness in children. The father returned home safely but the boy's brain did not come to a settlement. He continued to be sick until we treated him for his fear related to the particular incident.

Case Study: Dust Allergy Caused My Cough!

I suffered from chronic, irritable, nonproductive cough for five years, ever since I moved into the new house. I only coughed in the house or if I visited any dusty areas. My NAET practitioner asked me to collect house dust to bring in to her for treatment. I vacuumed the whole house including the carpet, corners of the rooms, sofa, drapes, etc., and took a random sample from the vacuum cleaner to the doctor. She treated me with NAET for the dust mix along with my own sample from the house. I was asked to stay away from my home for 25 hours. After 25 hours, when I returned to my home, I noticed that my five-year-old cough had left me. It hasn't returned in three years. Not only that, I don't cough if I visit any dusty places anymore. NAET is Great!

Bill Allen
Orange, California

Case Study: Asthma from Cleaning Agents

Marina 28, cleaned houses for a living. She had suffered from severe asthma ever since she began working. She was on three different medications to keep her asthma under control. Often she had to go to the emergency room when her asthma got severe. One of her friends gave her a copy of the Spanish edition of the book, "Say Good-bye to Illness." She immediately decided to try NAET. After she was treated for the NAET basics, she was treated for chemical mix and two other combinations: chemicals with

D.N.A, and Chemical mix with heat. Soon after those treatments, she was free from her asthma. Her asthma hasn't returned in four years.

Case Study: Fern Tree Caused His Seizures

Karl, a man in his early 60's, came to my office, nearly incapacitated by lapses of memory and seizures that resembled some form of epilepsy, Alzheimer's disease or perhaps a mild stroke. He would often wander off in total confusion or complete amnesia, sometimes losing track of significant blocks of time. Neurological examination and a CAT scan showed his brain-wave pattern to be completely normal. After considerable detective work, the cause in this case turned out to be the airborne spores of a fern tree he had recently planted in his backyard. After successful NAET treatment for the fern, his symptoms subsided.

Case Study: Knee Pains Caused by His Medication

Steven, a 43-year-old physical therapist, suffered from pain and swelling of both knees for over 3 months. Arthritis was suspected. His laboratory tests were normal for ANA. MRI did not reveal any abnormality of the knees. He did physical therapy on his knees regularly. It gave him temporary relief for an hour or so and then the pain returned and stayed with him for the rest of the day. He did not sleep more than half-an-hour at a time due to pain. He was taking pain pills every four hours. He had to be on disability. Then one day, while he was checking various web sites on pain management, he found the NAET website. He called for an appointment and came in. He was tested for allergies and found to be allergic to the prescription pills he was taking for his slightly elevated cholesterol. Since he lived a few minutes distance from our clinic, he was sent home to bring the pill. After successful NAET treatment for the cholesterol reducing pill, after approximately 45 minutes, he walked away without any knee pain.

He still had the swelling when he left the office. But on the following visit, his knees looked absolutely normal.

Case Study: Multiple Sclerosis

Crystal, a 24-year-old woman, was diagnosed as having multiple sclerosis. She had the typical symptoms of multiple sclerosis, numb hands, frequent headaches, lack of strength in both arms, extreme fatigue, shaking, weakness of the lower limbs, etc. She had been on a diet to lose weight for six months, which was when her symptoms started. During this time, she consumed lots of artificial sweeteners to which she was found to be highly allergic. When she was treated by NAET for artificial sweeteners, these symptoms disappeared.

Case Study: Potato and Breast Abscess

Jane, 24, came in complaining of bilateral breast abscesses over a period of three days. She had severe pain and could not wear normal clothes due to swelling and pain. She had eaten mashed potatoes, and potato chips four days in a row before she developed the pain and swelling of the breast. She was treated for potato by NAET immediately. She felt 60% better soon after the treatment. She needed two more treatments every ten minutes before she was sent home to rest. At the end of two days her breasts became normal. Amazingly, the body healed itself by disposing of the redness, pus-filled boils, and the painful abscess.

Case Study: Skin Rashes

For decades, I had a severe diffuse skin rash on my chest and upper abdomen due to allergies. After 8 months of weekly NAET treatments for food allergies, the skin rash disappeared.

Aladar Kabok, M.D.
NewPort Beach, California

Case Study: Weight Loss After Vitamin C Treatment

Michelle 37, had a height of 5 feet, 4 inches and weighed 218 pounds. She had weight problem all her life. She had tried different diets through the years. Finally she gave up on all diets, began eating vegetables and fruits only. Even with this restricted diet for months, she kept gaining more pounds. She retained water, had swollen ankles, shortness of breath, severe body aches, and suffered from frequent frontal headaches. She developed severe sinus problems and couldn't breathe through her nose due to blocked nostrils. She was referred to NAET by her family doctor. After three NAET basic treatments, she was treated for vitamin C. When she returned to the office after a week, she had lost 40 pounds. She was able to breathe normally, and had no more headaches. Her body aches had diminished greatly.

Case Study: Milk Allergy

As a small child, our son Andrew was sickly. He had tubes surgically inserted in his ears at age 4. Soon afterward he developed problems when he ate foods containing milk or chocolate. Andrew threw up his food, then was ravenously hungry afterward. Sometimes Andrew would suffer excruciating headaches as well. After many NAET treatments, Andrew began to improve. He was treated for the Basic 10 allergies, grains, chocolate, caffeine, milk, cheese, meat mix, heat, amino acids, leather and with many combinations.

Now Andrew is a healthy thirteen-year-old teenager, suffering an occasional headache instead of several headaches per week. I am cooking with regular milk now instead of rice milk and Andrew seems to tolerate it well.

Thank you, Dr. Devi, for your unfailing enthusiasm, which is apparent in your book, Say Good-bye to Illness. I know many families such as ours will be able to eat and function normally.

Karen Hyatt
Monroe, North Carolina

Case Study: Crohn's Disease

I almost lost my life. I was suffering from an extremely debilitating disease known as "Crohn's Disease." I was in and out of the hospital - and as every Crohn's patient discovers - treatment (other than surgical interventions), becomes large doses of prednisone (steroids) or other immunosuppressant drugs that are very harmful to the entire system. Also, once given a high dose, patients find it extremely difficult to stop taking them. NAET saved my life. Prednisone or other immunosuppressants may save the life of a patient if the patient is bleeding or starving to death because of the disease. However, the administration of the dangerous immunosuppressants to address the symptoms, is the only choice, since the real CAUSE of the disease is not yet known to the Western medicine.

Thank you Dr. Devi for giving me a NEW LIFE! Dr. Devi Nambudripad's NAET treatments addressed the CAUSE of Crohn's Disease. I was allergic to all NAET basic groups, some of my own body tissues (small and large bowels, mucous membrane, parasites and blood) as well as some bacteria causing inflammation. After I was treated successfully for the above allergens, I started feeling better. My ongoing struggle to lower the dosage of prednisone had been frustrated at 35 milligrams. Then, after just a few treatments of NAET, I was able to drop the dose from 35 mg to 5 mg with no adverse affects. Eventually, I was able to stop it altogether. There were no symptoms of bleeding or starvation or relapse of the disease.

I will not face any future surgical procedure, or lose any part of my intestine.

Thank you, from the bottom of my heart, Dr. Nambudripad, for discovering the cure for such serious illnesses as "Crohn's Disease."

Cathy Carlson, Buena Park, CA
After five years, Cathy still remains free of any previous symptoms of Crohn's Disease and leading a normal life.

Case Study: Bed Linen Linked to Sciatic Pain

Genine, a 56-year-old hospital clerk suffered from sciatic pain for 11 months. She was getting treated in the same hospital where she worked for many years. She took pain medications, did physical therapy, took warm baths, with no improvement. She felt worse at night. She could hardly sleep during the night. She lived alone and was frustrated with this nagging pain. Finally, she was referred to us by her treating physician for acupuncture treatments. In our office she was tested and found that she was allergic to her bed linen, blanket, a pair of shoes, and a pair of slippers, all bought about a year ago for Christmas. She wore the shoes daily to work and the slippers she wore when she returned from work. Then she slept in the bed with the bed linen and blanket. Ever since she began using the bed linen and blanket, she began experiencing sciatic pain. So she did not take time to wash the clothes or change the sheets. She couldn't go out, had no social life the last year. Her friend drove her to work and back. Even though she had constant pains, she managed to sit and do the clerical job at the nurses station. When she was treated for the shoes, slippers and bed linen, she was freed from the sciatic pain. She was also treated for all the basics to insure better health in the future.

Case Study: Allergy to Pet Caused Eczema

We found NAET as an answer to my second daughter's eczema. Within 3 early treatments Lianna's eczema had gone from a bleeding rash covering most of her body to an occasional redness behind her knees. I had also been having treatments for lifelong allergies and we were both enjoying the freedom that comes with NAET.

That was until her new pets arrived, a rabbit and guinea pig that she didn't put down for days. Lianna's discomfort began showing up as restless nights and I was itching and couldn't sleep. On the third night after the animals arrived home, Lianna woke up at 10 pm crying, hot and itching, with inflamed eyes and a runny nose. I undressed her and she was covered in an eczema rash.

We were having dinner with friends, one of whom happened to be qualified in NAET. Lianna and I were both allergic to the new pets and she treated us then and there. We both slept well that night, Lianna's symptoms resolved and the rash receded over the next few days and I stopped itching. Since then the animals are kissed and cuddled everyday without any problem.

This is just one of many NAET treatments I can be thankful for. Thanks Devi and the NAET practitioners who have helped us here in Melbourne.

Lisa Bodley
Victoria, Australia

Case Study: Breast Cancer Caused from Allergies

A 64 year-college professor was diagnosed with adenocarcinoma, a type of breast cancer. She had a plum size self-contained tumor. Surgery was suggested. She wanted to try alternative treatments before she consented for surgery. She approached us for NAET. Her family members had benefited from NAET for various allergy-related disorders. She was found to be allergic to potato, coffee, lima beans, milk products, bra, deodorant, dry cleaning chemicals and hormone progesterone. After she was treated for all these, her biopsy was repeated by her oncologist and found negative for cancer.

NAET can help only allergy-related cancers.

Case Study: Allergic to Newspaper Ink

Will, 49, complained of severe pains in the right elbow, the wrist joint and the first interphalangeal joints. He had been treated for carpal tunnel syndrome, tenosynovitis, and tennis elbow many times before he came to us. When he was evaluated in our office, he was found to be highly allergic to paper, one of the tools of his trade as a writer. His symptoms cleared up soon after he was treated successfully with NAET.

Case Study: Headaches

An example of a paper allergy was observed during an interview with an attorney, who complained that he always came away from his office with a headache and feeling so tired that he could only go home and immediately go to bed. This attorney was allergic to paper, with a completely different reaction from that of the writer.

Case Study: Severe Reaction to Bee Sting

In 1986, I was traveling in England when I was stung by a bee on my left arm. I was treated with an antihistamine and an antibiotic. My arm grew steadily worse, I flew home in that condition, thinking that it would heal in time. Nine days later, I was entertaining a slight fever in my arm and unusual redness. It had become more swollen than ever and more uncomfortable.

My friend insisted I visit Dr. Devi. I was afraid of acupuncture. I had little knowledge of it. Vision of needles in my body was also unpleasant. If antibiotics could not help, what could she do? In desperation, I allowed her to take me to her office. I found Dr. Devi interesting and knowledgeable and her profound confidence that she could help me right then persuaded me to let her treat me. I found the treatment relaxing and even enjoyable. I could not believe that the needles did not hurt - almost immediately I felt better. By morning, after the best night's rest I had experienced in days, I found the swelling was gone! Was this my arm? It sure was! I called her and said, " It is a miracle, I am coming back today." Since that time she has treated me for all my allergies. I feel now I am "allergy free."

Ileen Coons
Fullerton, Calif.

Case Study: Reaction to DPT Immunization

A four-year-old boy became very sick after a regular DPT immunization. He had continuous fever (102 degrees Fahrenheit) for six weeks. Finally, when the fever came down to a normal level, he had a dull response to everyday activities. He became normal after he was treated for DPT.

Case Study: Reaction to Small Pox Vaccination

Phil, 42, was referred to us by one of his friends who was also our patient. Phil had experienced weakness of his right leg for 35 years. He could not take part in sports activities in school while he was growing up. When he was in his early teens, he began experiencing the symptoms of irritable bowels. With all these health problems, he stopped his education soon after he graduated from high school. He found a clerical job in the city hall, got married and had two children. His irritable bowels continued to bother him on and off. When it flared up he had to stay home on a milk diet. Milk seemed to soothe his pain in the abdomen. In our office, NTT (Nambudripad's testing techniques, read Chapter 3 for more information on NTT) revealed that his leg weakness and the irritable bowels started after the small pox vaccination he received in primary school. After the NAET basics, he was successfully treated for small pox vaccination and his right leg became normal once again. He continued with the irritable bowel syndrome until he was treated for grains, heat and small pox vaccination as a combination. None of his previous symptoms have returned in four years.

Case Study: Canker Sores

One of the young patients who came to our office had a history of canker sores whenever he walked in the sun. He was highly allergic to vitamin D, one of the vitamins produced in the body with the help of sunlight. After he was treated by NAET for vitamin D, the incidents of canker sores as a result of walking in the sun diminished.

Case Study: Allergy to Cold

Helene, 74, liked to drink cold water, but she always choked on icy cold water. She also developed an allergic dry cough whenever she ate ice cream. She was treated for all the ingredients in the ice cream, yet her coughing spells and choking incidents persisted. She was finally treated for actual ice cubes. Afterwards, she could enjoy ice water and ice cream without choking.

Case Study: Raynaud's Disease

Jenny, 58, suffered from Raynaud's Disease. The tip of her fingers remained dark blue on a cold day. She was allergic to cold, citrus fruits, and meat products. She felt better when she was cleared for the above items.

Case Study: Skin Cancer

Michael, 32, who frequently had skin cancer on his face, was evaluated and found to be highly allergic to the stainless steel blade of the razor he used. The use of a popular skin cream was the cause of the beginning of skin cancer in another patient. She was allergic to vitamin A and to the skin cream itself. After she was treated for these substances, her lesions cleared up.

Case Study: Bronchial Asthma

A woman who suffered from bronchial asthma was cleared of her asthma when she was treated for pneumococcus, the bacterium responsible for pneumonia. Both of her parents had died of pneumonia soon after her birth.

Case Study: Chronic Bronchitis

Ray, a man of 44, responded well to the treatment for diphtheria, thus clearing his chronic bronchitis. He had inherited the tendency toward allergies from his mother, who almost died from diphtheria when she was seven. The reaction to diphtheria was manifested in him as bronchitis, sinusitis and arthritis.

Case Study: Epstein-Barr Virus

Jill, 55, suffered from the Epstein-Barr virus and various allergies. After treatment for the virus, her response was very encouraging. Upon questioning her, it was found that her Japanese parents, uncles and aunts died of tuberculosis. She was immediately tested and treated for tuberculosis and she became allergy free and healthy once again.

Case Study: Migraines

Sara, 42, had severe migraines all her life. Her mother had rheumatic fever as a child. Treatment for rheumatic fever lessened her migraines.

Case Study: An Allergy to Cotton Socks

Mike 31, came to the clinic for treatment of athlete's foot. In the interview he disclosed that he has suffered from athlete's foot for years. He was unsuccessful to help his feet using numerous treatments that he had tried for years. The infection was not only distracting and painful, but was also destroying his toenails. The problem was increasing to the point that it started to interfere with his passion for tennis. During allergy testing, it was discovered that he was allergic to the cotton in his socks. He also mentioned that he dried his feet with cotton towels. After treatment for cotton, his athlete's foot cleared up.

Case Study: 32 Surgeries in 28 years

Such was the story of Nancy, 28-years old, when she came to our office with complaints of severe migraine headaches. She suffered these headaches nearly once a week, which kept her in bed on medications. Also, she was frequently given pain shots. On examination of her history, we learned that she vomited every meal as an infant and when she was a child. She had 32 surgeries during her 28 years. This included a hernia surgery when she was an infant, seven surgeries for gastric ulcers, six for her knees, two for her nose and two for her sinuses. She also had four surgeries on her shoulders, one to remove a cyst from her ovary, two on her ankle, two for the bladder, one for the ear and one for the throat to remove her tonsils. She had the feeling of a big mass on one side of her head whenever she had a migraine. Brain swelling was the cause of this so called mass. Finally, she was advised to have brain surgery to prevent the severe debilitating migraine, when a friend referred her to us.

Muscle response testing revealed that she was highly allergic to almost every substance around her including food, drinks, clothing, carpet, bed linen, and her pets. She was treated by NAET for nearly a year, at the rate of five treatments a week, for all the basics, and every item she came in contact with in her everyday life. For the first few treatments, we concentrated on her regular food items. Then she was treated for her clothing, cosmetics, etc. By the end of three months, her migraines became less frequent and less intense. At the end of one year, she could almost live a normal life, not a life ruled by her sicknesses. If her parents had learned MRT to test allergies, she wouldn't have had 32 surgeries in her 28 years.

Incidentally, toward the end of the treatments, she met a young man and fell in love for the first time in her life. A year later, they got married. This is one of many happy endings to an otherwise miserable situation.

Case Study: Hives From Birth

Let's look at the history of six-year-old Ray, who suffered severe allergies from birth. On the second day of his life, he developed red, angry-looking hives all over his body. He began spitting up every meal, whether it was water or milk. He suffered from severe constipation, insomnia, irritability, colic pains and severe eczema. When he was six months old, his pediatrician suggested purse-string surgery (tightening up the lower segment of the esophagus to prevent continuous vomiting). But he was luckier than Nancy. His mother had learned MRT and tested everything before she gave it to him. She fed him only non-allergic food items every day for four years (Cream of rice cereal, nonfat Carnation dry milk and water). He did fairly well on the special diet. His eczema was under control. He slept better. His constipation was relieved. His colic pain diminished. He appeared happy and friendly. When he was four, he began treatment through NAET. In a year or so, after being treated for various allergies, he was able to eat normal food and was ready for school. He is a healthy teenager now.

Case Study: Chinese Food Triggered Asthma

Tina, a nine-year-old girl, was undergoing treatment for asthma by NAET. She was treated for various foods and was able to eat all of them without provoking an asthmatic attack. One day, her parents took her to a Chinese restaurant. When the food was brought to the table, she immediately whispered to her mother that she thought she was allergic to some of the food items on the plate and that she might become ill if she ate them. The girl's mother ignored her and forced her to eat the food, saying that she had been treated for all of them. Before she finished eating, she had an asthmatic attack. The confused mother brought a sample of everything the child ate to the office the next day. She was found to be allergic to the mixed vegetables that contained a great deal of cornstarch. She had not yet been treated for the corn. The nine-year-old was able to recognize the allergen before she ate it. She said her throat started itching as soon as the food was placed in front of her, giving her a clue that she might be allergic to something on the plate.

Case Study: Sciatic Neuralgia

John, 32, a single man with no immediate family, suffered from severe right sided sciatic pain and neuralgia for 14 years. His pains felt somewhat better at night towards morning, but as the day progressed, he felt miserable. He was examined, evaluated, X-rayed, scanned, by various specialists. All tests including laboratory tests looked normal in all areas. His tests were repeated many times and found negative repeatedly. He took different pain medications given by different medical practitioners. He tried chiropractic treatments, acupuncture treatments, massages, detoxification programs, nutritional program and even psychological counseling over the years without much relief. Finally he believed that he suffered from some "mysterious, incurable" disorder. He worked as an automobile sales person and somehow by clenching his teeth he managed to keep his job. Then, after suffering for fourteen years, he was referred to us by one of his family friends who had just discovered NAET. He had no hope when he came to see me. Later he told us that he came in just to please his friend. In our office he was evaluated and found John was actually one of the healthy ones we rarely get to meet. Our office is known to get all "last resort patients" who would be allergic to everything under the sun. But John surprised us. He did not have too many food or environmental allergies. But, he was found to be allergic to his leather shoes and walking shoes. He was immediately treated for his leather shoes which he wears every day to work as a salesman.

On the following visit, he reported that his pain was 80% relieved. On the second visit, he tested non-allergic to his leather shoes and was treated for his walking shoe. On the third visit, he was still allergic to the walking shoes and we found that the shoelace was still the problem. Shoelaces are made with a different material than the shoes themselves. After he was treated for the laces, he was completely relieved of his fourteen-year-old leg pain.

Case Study: Allergic to Pasta Caused his Eczema

I have a five-year-old patient with eczema and skin rashes who can test his allergies to foods in his way more accurately than his mother's MRT test on him. One day his mother tested him on his pasta dinner and found him to be non-allergic to it. But he insisted that he was allergic to the pasta not the sauce. Due to the mother's insistence, he ate the pasta and woke up in hives and rashes in the morning. The mother brought him to the office and I found him to be allergic to the pasta and not the tomato sauce. Then his mother told me that he intuitively knew it before he ate it. So he told me that he held a piece of pasta in his hand and he felt tingling all over as if he was being tickled by someone. He had learned the testing procedure at one of our patient-education seminars. He paid attention and learned it but not the mother.

When he completed his treatment for pasta and grains, his eczema and rashes cleared up.

Case Study: Allergy to Cotton

A 28-year-old woman was treated for cotton. After seven consecutive treatments, she decided to go on a short vacation before being cleared of her allergy, without informing her allergist. Three months later, her husband called and asked whether NAET could help his wife's present condition. Two days into her vacation, she had slipped into a depression and refused to talk or cooperate with anyone. As a teenager, she had experienced a nervous breakdown but recovered completely. Finally, the husband took her to two psychotherapists, neither of whom could help her out of the depression. The allergist remembered that she had not completed treatment for cotton. She was brought into the office and treated for cotton and was cleared after four more treatments, a total of eleven. At the end of these treatments, she came out of her depression.

Case Study: Can Allergies Cause Miscarriage?

A 22-year-old woman who had two miscarriages came to our office. We found that she was allergic to most of the foods she was eating. She was treated for most of the allergies, but then she got pregnant again and discontinued the treatments. This time she carried full term and had a normal child. She returned again, to treat for herself, as well as for the child. When the child was examined, we discovered he was not allergic to the items the mother had passed before she got pregnant; however, he was allergic to the items the mother had not yet treated.

Case Study: An Allergy to Fabrics Caused Skin rashes

A young couple, both of whom manifested a number of allergic problems, including migraines, dizzy spells, sinusitis, joint pains etc., were treated for all their known allergies. Then they had a child. We checked the child and found that the child was absolutely healthy with no known allergies at all. Another couple, both allergic to many items, were treated for all the foods, but did not get treated for any fabrics. When their child was born, she developed severe rashes all over her body and could not wear any clothes. The parents brought the child in for evaluation, and we found she was allergic to all the fabrics, but not to the food items.

Case Study: Artichoke and Backaches

Artichoke seems to be a simple vegetable, but it has created many different types of pain disorders in a great number of my patients. A young man of 22 came in with a two-month history of severe, acute pain in his right lateral thigh, radiating into the right knee and ankle joint. During NTT evaluation, it was discovered that he was reacting to the artichoke he ate 2 months earlier. He never liked artichoke, but was at a party where he was served artichoke. The next morning he woke up with sciatic pain on his right thigh. He tried various treatments before he discovered NAET. His pain got worse in spite of all the pain pills he consumed. He stopped working and had to go on temporary disability. After the evaluation, I treated him for artichoke. His gallbladder and colon were blocked. Eighty percent of his sciatic pain was relieved almost instantly. After 12 minutes, he was completely free of his pain.

Case Study: An allergy to Vitamin C

Carmel was getting treated by one of the NAET practitioners for constant, severe pain in her liver and spleen. None of the tests showed any abnormalities. When she was evaluated by an NAET practitioner, she was found to be allergic to many allergen groups except the vitamin C group. She continued the treatments with him for two years. Her condition did not improve. Finally, the practitioner sent her to me for evaluation. She was found to be highly allergic to vitamin C. Within 30 minutes of her treatment for vitamin C, she reported that the pain in her liver and spleen was relieved completely. Had the practitioner tested the patient properly, had he found the weakness on Vitamin C group, had he treated her for vitamin C, she would have been free of pain after the fourth NAET treatment instead of suffering for two years.

Case Study: Chronic Low Back Pain

I suffered from low back pain for years. I have tried other treatments for the same pain in the past without any result. Then I started NAET. I received several NAET treatments for the pain to no avail. Devi's tests indicated that the water I was drinking was a main source of the pain. According to her the water chemicals were affecting my liver and gall bladder. But I had to wait until I completed Minerals and salt mix treatment before treating for the water chemicals.

During one of Mala's later treatments for the left, lower back pain, I asked Mala why the pain moved from my left knee to my left back, hip and leg. Then she said something most significant. She said because both locations are on the gall bladder meridian. This gave us the idea to treat the entire gall bladder meridian. MRT was also weak on Urinary bladder meridian. She treated me for the gall bladder and urinary bladder tissue in the office. Then I continued to self-treat every two hours at home. I then self-treated a combo of the bladder tissue with my drinking water. Then I treated a combo of the bladder tissue, gall bladder tissue, liver tissue and water. END OF PAIN 100% !

Now all my meridians are unblocked and clear and I feel really young and strong. Without both Devi and Mala—the dynamic duo—and without the skills they taught me, I never would have found the sources of the pain, treated them and eliminated them 100%.

Dikran Ayarian, Ph.D
Beverly Hills, California

Case Study: Vulvodynia

I am very happy to report to you that I am completely free of my vulvodynia over a year now. I am very thankful to you and NAET for helping me to be free from my so called "Incurable Disorder." I wanted to tell you that I've been referring people to the NAET website. Last fall when I was having all of that pain during intercourse and after, I registered with the vulvodynia support network. I have recently been getting a lot of contacts wanting to know what NAET was and how it helped me. Vulvodynia was what I was diagnosed with from the doctors here. Unfortunately there are many many women diagnosed with this as well and there is no "cure" and many treatments don't work well and have awful side effects. So I have been posting messages on the vulvodynia websites about how NAET helped me. So hopefully some of these women will check it out in their area and maybe receive some relief and success in treating their "untreatable" condition. Just thought you'd want to know.

Brianne, New Mexico
NAET Sp of this patient: Marilyn Chernoff,
Albuquerque, New Mexico, (505) 292-2222

Case Study: Movement Caused My Back Pain

This letter is to thank you for the incredible results that I have experienced with NAET since starting treatments. The shifts in my body that have occurred from your treatments are amazing! My hair, my nails, my skin, everything looks and feels healthier and stronger as I am obviously retaining my nutrients. One of the treatments was just amazing! I had to have my sister help me walk into the office. I was in a slump position as if I had strained my back or had a spasm. I could barely move. I was in a lot of pain. Movement was unbearable. You diagnosed my problem as a movement disorder. Two days prior to my appointment, I had a session on a Chi Machine. The doctor left me on the table for thirty minutes, the normal session is no longer than 10 minutes. I was treated for the movement of a Chi Machine with the assistance of another person. After the 20 minutes on the table, I was able to walk out of the office and stand straighter than I had been able to five days prior! Your NAET treatments have changed my body, mind and soul for a healthier new year!!! The value of your treatments is immeasurable.

Sonya Sanchez
Albuquerque, New Mexico
NAET Sp of this patient: Marilyn Chernoff,
Albuquerque, New Mexico, (505) 292-2222

Liebshen's Story

At 3 A.M. on September 21, 2002, I rushed Liebshen, my Dachshund, to an emergency veterinary hospital. She had delivered puppies only six days before, and her breathing had become so rapid and loud as she nursed, that I was terrified we would lose her. After a full examination, blood work-up and X-Rays, I was told that she had chronic bronchitis, but worse still, a serious uterine infection.

They wanted to keep her, start IV's and prepare for surgery, although I was warned that she "might not make it." Her uterus was very large, and the breathing problem made the anesthesia situation difficult. Even if she survived the surgery, they doubted that she would be able to care for or nurse the puppies.

Although the doctor warned me that Liebshen might die, I could not leave her (and the four puppies) there. I felt that the psychological trauma would be too much for her to bear. So she was started on oral antibiotics and bronchial medications and we went home. The morning was stressful. Although her breathing improved slightly, she was strangely restless, and avoided nursing the puppies.

In the meantime, Dr. Devi Nambudripad had begun the first day of an NAET Self-Help Program at SKY Farm, which I was scheduled to attend. As I heard later, Dr. Devi was talking to the group about her experiences in treating both people and animals with NAET. Candace Smith, who was a student in the course, explained to Dr. Nambudripad that I had not come because of Liebshen's illness. Dr. Devi asked for details of the Dachshund's condition, and then agreed to visit her at the lunch break. All the attendees of the program which included doctors, psychologists, counselors, body workers and Yoga teachers, were very interested to see if NAET could help the dog.

While still at the seminar, Candace phoned me and put Dr. Devi on the line. She told me that she would come to see us during lunch break, and asked if there was anything new, any new liquid in Libshen's diet. Startled by the question, I had to think for a moment, then realized the answer was milk. She instructed that I not give the dog any more milk or milk products, and to put some of the same milk she had been drinking into a small glass jar. She also told me to collect some of the infected discharge from Liebshen's vagina, and put that in a jar too before her arrival at noon.

Two hours later, Dr. Devi arrived. We talked for a few minutes and then the NAET treatment began. Dr. Devi sat in a chair while I sat on the floor with my back in front of her legs and Liebshen on my lap. I held the milk jar next to the dog's body, while Dr. Devi did the testing and NAET on my back. As the surrogate, I did the specific breathing technique that she instructed me to do.

After the NAET process, Dr. Devi said that the milk allergy not only caused the respiratory crisis, but that it weakened the uterus. The childbirth had weakened it further and that was why the infection had developed.

When some time had passed, Dr. Devi did NAET with the discharge and then treated Liebshen for the emotions. She said afterward that Liebshen was grieving over the loss of the two puppies (one was stillborn, the other passed away at four days of age); she had no energy left to feed the litter, she was afraid she was going to die, and was distraught about what would happen to the babies when she was gone. But Dr. Devi assured me that now Liebshen knew she would be O.K.

Before leaving, Dr. Devi taught me the follow-up treatment to give Liebshen several times throughout the rest of the day and evening. She said that although my dog was very sick, she believed that Liebshen would recover. She felt that an operation would not be necessary; that Liebshen would pass the material naturally. And she thought that her lungs would be O.K.

Within minutes of Dr. Devi's leaving, Liebshen went into the whelping box and began feeding the puppies. Her breathing that night was far better, and her overall condition seemed much improved.

The next morning, my regular veterinary clinic was open. The vet had been faxed all the information from the emergency hospital. Liebshen had a full examination, including ultrasound. To my utter amazement, the doctor said that Liebshen did not have bronchitis, just some mild respiratory congestion. He also said that her uterus was shrinking nicely, postpartum. He prescribed one week of antibiotics, and gave me bronchial medications "just in case." He said to phone him in one week, but that he would not have to see her again unless she had some difficulty. I went home in a daze.

Liebshen completed the antibiotics without a problem. I never had to give her any bronchial medication. She is doing great. The puppies are doing great.

Miracle is not a word to be used lightly. But it is the only word that is appropriate for Liebshen's story. Thank you Dr. Devi. May God bless you and your work.

Barbara Levitt
Philadelphia

GLOSSARY

Acetaldehyde: An aldehyde found in cigarette smoke, vehicle exhaust, and smog. It is a metabolic product of Candida Albicans and is synthesized from alcohol in the liver.

Acetylcholine: A neurotransmitter manufactured in the brain, used for memory and control of sensory input and muscular output signals.

Acid: Any compound capable of releasing a hydrogen ion; its pH value will be less than 7.

Acute: Extremely sharp or severe, as in pain. Can also refer to an illness or reaction that is sudden and intense.

Adaptation: Ability of an organism to integrate new elements into its environment.

Addiction: A dependent state characterized by cravings for a particular substance if that substance is withdrawn.

Additive: A substance added in small amounts to foods to alter the food in some way.

Adrenaline: Trademark for preparations of epinephrine, which is a hormone secreted by the adrenal gland. It is used sublingually and by injection to stop allergic reactions.

Aldehyde: A class of organic compounds obtained by oxidation of alcohol. Formaldehyde and acetaldehyde are members of this class of compounds.

Alkaline: Basic, or any substance that accepts a hydrogen ion; its pH value will be greater than 7.

Allergenic: Causing or producing an allergic reaction.

Allergen: Any organic or inorganic substance from one's surroundings or from within the body itself that causes an allergic response in an individual is called an allergen. An allergen can cause an IgE antibody mediated or non-IgE mediated response in a person. Some of the commonly known allergens are: pollens, molds, animal dander, food and drinks, chemicals of a different kind like the ones found in food, water, air, fabrics, cleaning agents, environmental materials, detergent, make-up products etc., body secretions, bacteria, virus, synthetic materials, fumes, and air pollution. Emotional unpleasant thoughts like anger, frustration, etc., can also become allergens and cause allergic reactions in people.

Allergic reaction: Adverse, varied symptoms, unique to each person, resulting from the body's response to exposure to allergens.

Allergic shiners: Dark circles under the eyes, usually indicative of allergies.

Allergy: Attacks by the immune system on harmless or even useful things entering the body. Abnormal responses to substances usually well tolerated by most people.

Amino acid: An organic acid that contains an amino (ammonia-like NH3) chemical group; the building blocks that make up all proteins.

Anaphylactic shock: Also known as anaphylaxis. Usually it happens suddenly when exposed to a highly allergic item; but sometimes, it can also happen as a cumulative reaction. (The first two doses of penicillin may not trigger a severe reaction, but the third or fourth one could produce an anaphylaxis in some people). An anaphylaxis (a life-threatening allergic reaction) is characterized by: An immediate allergic reaction that can cause difficulty in breathing, lightheadedness, fainting, chills, internal cold, severe heart palpitation or irregular heart beat, pallor, eyes rolling, poor mental clarity, tremors, internal shaking, extreme fear, angio-neurotic edema, throat swelling, drop in blood pressure, nausea, vomiting, diarrhea, swelling anywhere in the body, redness and hives, fever, delirium, unresponsiveness, or sometimes even death.

Antibody: A protein molecule produced in the body by lymphocytes in response to a perceived harmful foreign or abnormal substance (another protein) as a defense mechanism to protect the body.

Antigen: Any substance recognized by the immune system that causes the body to produce antibodies; also refers to a concentrated solution of an allergen.

Antihistamine: A chemical that blocks the reaction of histamine that is released by the mast cells and basophils during an allergic reaction. Any substance that slows oxidation, prevents damage from free radicals and results in oxygen sparing.

Assimilate: To incorporate into a system of the body; to transform nutrients into living tissue.

Autoimmune: A condition resulting when the body makes antibodies against its own tissues or fluid. The immune system attacks the body it inhabits, which causes damage or alteration of cell function.

Basophils: A type of white blood cell that mediates inflammatory reactions. They are functionally similar to mast cells and are found in mucous membranes, skin, and bronchial tubes.

B-cell: A white blood cell. It produces antibodies as directed by the T-cells.

Binder: A substance added to tablets to help hold them together.

Blood brain barrier: A cellular barrier that prevents certain chemicals from passing from the blood to the brain.

Buffer: A substance that minimizes changes in pH (acidity or alkalinity).

Candida albicans: A genus of yeast-like fungi normally found in the body. It can multiply and often cause severe infections, allergic reactions or toxicity.

Candidiasis: An overgrowth of Candida organisms, which are part of the normal flora of the mouth, skin, intestines and vagina.

Carbohydrate, complex: Two molecules of sugar linked together, found in whole grains, vegetables, and fruits. This metabolizes into glucose slower than refined carbohydrate.

Carbohydrate, refined: A molecule of sugar that metabolizes quickly into glucose, e.g., white flour, white sugar, and white rice.

Catalyst: A chemical that speeds up a chemical reaction without being consumed or permanently affected in the process.

Cerebral allergy: Mental dysfunction caused by sensitivity to foods, chemicals, environmental substances, or other substances like work materials etc.

Chronic: Of long duration.

Chronic fatigue syndrome: A syndrome of multiple symptoms most commonly associated with fatigue and reduced energy or no energy.

Crohn's disease: An intestinal disorder associated with irritable bowel syndrome, inflammation of the bowels and colitis.

Cumulative reaction: A type of reaction caused by an accumulation of allergens in the body.

Cyclic allergy: A type of allergy which will disappear and will not reappear unless there is overexposure to the substance.

Cytokine: A chemical produced by the T-cells during an infection as our immune system's second line of defense. Examples of cytokines are interleukin 2 and gamma interferon.

Desensitization: The process of building up body tolerance to allergens by the use of extracts of the allergenic substance.

Detoxification: A variety of methods used to reduce toxic materials accumulated in body tissues.

Digestive tract: Includes the salivary glands, mouth, esophagus, stomach, small intestine, portions of the liver, pancreas, and large intestine.

Disorder: A disturbance of regular or normal functions.

Dust: Dust particles from various sources irritate sensitive individuals, causing different respiratory problems like asthma, bronchitis, hay fever-like symptoms, sinusitis, and cough.

Dust mites: Microscopic insects that live in dusty areas, pillows, blankets, bedding, carpets, upholstered furniture, drapes, corners of the houses where people neglect to clean regularly.

Eczema: An inflammatory process of the skin resulting from skin allergies causing dry, itchy, crusty, scaly, weepy, blisters or eruptions on the skin. Skin rash frequently caused by allergy.

Edema: Excess fluid accumulation in tissue spaces. It could be localized or generalized.

Electromagnetic: Refers to emissions and interactions of both electric and magnetic components. Magnetism arising from electric charge in motion. This has a definite amount of energy.

Elimination diet: A diet in which common allergenic foods and those suspected of causing allergic symptoms have been temporarily eliminated.

Endocrine: Refers to ductless glands that manufacture and secrete hormones into the blood stream or extracellular fluids.

Endocrine system: Thyroid, parathyroid, pituitary, hypothalamus, adrenal glands, pineal gland, gonads, the intestinal tract, kidneys, liver, and placenta.

Endogenous: Originating from or due to internal causes.

Environment: A total of circumstances and/or surroundings in which an organism exists. May be a combination of internal or external influences that can affect an individual.

Environmental illness: A complex set of symptoms caused by adverse reactions of the body to external and internal environments.

Enzyme: A substance, usually protein in nature and formed in living cells, which starts or stops biochemical reactions.

Eosinophil: A type of white blood cell. Eosinophil levels may be high in some cases of allergy or parasitic infestation.

Erythrocyte: Red blood cell.

Exocrine: Refers to substance released through ducts that lead to a body compartment or surface.

Exogenous: Originating from or due to external causes.

Extracellular: Situated outside a cell or cells.

Extract: Treatment dilution of an antigen used in immunotherapy, such as food, chemical, or pollen extract.

Fibromyalgia: An immune complex disorder causing general body aches, muscle aches, and general fatigue.

Fight or flight: The activation of the sympathetic branch of the autonomic nervous system, preparing the body to meet a threat or challenge.

Food addiction: A person becomes dependent on a particular allergenic food and must keep eating it regularly in order to prevent withdrawal symptoms.

Food grouping: A grouping of foods according to their botanical or biological characteristics.

Free radical: A substance with unpaired electrons, which is attracted to cell membranes and enzymes where it binds and causes damage.

Gastrointestinal: Relating both to stomach and intestines.

Heparin: A substance released during allergic reaction. Heparin has anti-inflammatory action in the body.

Histamine: A body substance released by mast cells and basophils during allergic reactions, which precipitates allergic symptoms.

Holistic: Refers to the idea that health and wellness depend on a balance between physical (structural) aspects, physiological (chemical, nutritional, functional) aspects, emotional and spiritual aspects of a person.

Homeopathic: Refers to giving minute amounts of remedies that in massive doses would produce effects similar to the condition being treated.

Homeostasis: A state of perfect balance in the organism also called Yin-Yang balance. The balance of functions and chemical composition within an organism that results from the actions of regulatory systems.

Hormone: A chemical substance that is produced in the body, secreted into body fluids, and is transported to other organs, where it produces a specific effect on metabolism.

Hydrocarbon: A chemical compound that contains only hydrogen and carbon.

Hypersensitivity: An acquired reactivity to an antigen that can result in bodily damage upon subsequent exposure to that particular antigen.

Hyperthyroidism: A condition resulting from over-function of the thyroid gland.

Hypoallergenic: Refers to products formulated to contain the minimum possible allergens: some people with few allergies can tolerate them well. Severely allergic people can still react to these items.

Hypothyroidism: A condition resulting from under-function of the thyroid gland.

IgA: Immunoglobulin A, an antibody found in secretions associated with mucous membranes.

IgD: Immunoglobulin D, an antibody found on the surface of B-cells.

IgE: Immunoglobulin E, an antibody responsible for immediate hypersensitivity and skin reactions.

IgG: Immunoglobulin G, also known as gammaglobulin, the major antibody in the blood that protects against bacteria and viruses.

IgM: Immunoglobulin M, the first antibody to appear during an immune response.

Immune system: The body's defense system, composed of specialized cells, organs, and body fluids. It has the ability to locate, neutralize, metabolize and eliminate unwanted or foreign substances.

Immunocompromised: A person whose immune system has been damaged or stressed and is not functioning properly.

Immunity: Inherited, acquired, or induced state of being, able to resist a particular antigen by producing antibodies to counteract it. A unique mechanism of the organism to protect and maintain its body against adversity in its surroundings.

Inflammation: The reaction of tissues to injury from trauma, infection, or irritating substances. Affected tissue can be hot, reddened, swollen, and tender.

Inhalant: Any airborne substance small enough to be inhaled into the lungs; eg., pollen, dust, mold, animal danders, perfume, smoke, and smell from chemical compounds.

Intolerance: Inability of an organism to utilize a substance.

Intracellular: Situated within a cell or cells.

Intradermal: Method of testing in which a measured amount of antigen is injected between the top layers of the skin.

Ion: An atom that has lost or gained an electron and thus carries an electric charge.

Kinesiology: Science of movement of the muscle.

Latent: Concealed or inactive.

Leukocytes: White blood cells.

Lipids: Fats and oils that are insoluble in water. Oils are liquids in room temperature and fats are solid.

Lymph: A clear, watery, alkaline body fluid found in the lymph vessels and tissue spaces. Contains mostly white blood cells.

Lymphocyte: A type of white blood cell, usually classified as T-or B-cells.

Macrophage: A white blood cell that kills and ingests microorganisms and other body cells.

Masking: Suppression of symptoms due to frequent exposure to a substance to which a person is sensitive.

Mast cells: Large cells containing histamine, found in mucous membranes and skin cells. The histamine in these cells is released during certain allergic reactions.

Mediated: Serving as the vehicle to bring about a phenomenon. For example, an IgE-mediated reaction is one in which IgE changes cause the symptoms and the reaction to proceed.

Membrane: A thin sheet or layer of pliable tissue that lines a cavity, connects two structures, selective barrier.

Metabolism: Complex chemical and electrical processes in living cells by which energy is produced and life is maintained. New material is assimilated for growth, repair, and replacement of tissues. Waste products are excreted.

Migraine: A condition marked by recurrent severe headaches, often on one side of the head, often accompanied by nausea, vomiting, and light aura. These headaches are frequently attributed to food allergy.

Mineral: An inorganic substance. The major minerals in the body are calcium, phosphorus, potassium, sulfur, sodium, chloride, and magnesium.

Monocyte: A type of white blood cell.

Mucous membranes: Moist tissues forming the lining of body cavities that have an external opening, such as the respiratory, digestive, and urinary tracts.

Muscle Response Testing: A testing technique based on kinesiology to test allergies by comparing the strength of a muscle or a group of muscles in the presence and absence of the allergen.

NAET: (Nambudripad's Allergy Elimination Techniques)**:** A technique to eliminate allergies permanently from the body towards the treated allergen. Developed by Dr. Devi S. Nambudripad in 1983 and practiced by over 4,500 medical practitioners worldwide. This technique is completely natural, non-invasive, and drug-free. It has been effectively used in treating all types of allergies and problems arising from allergies. It is taught by Dr. Nambudripad in Buena Park, CA to currently licensed medical practitioners. If you are interested and want to learn more about NAET or attend a seminar, please visit the website: www.naet.com.

Nervous system: A network made up of nerve cells, the brain, and the spinal cord, which regulates and coordinates body activities.

Neuro-transmitter: A molecule that transmits electrical and/or chemical messages from nerve cell (neuron) to nerve cell or from nerve cell to muscle, secretory, or organ cells.

Nutrients: Vitamins, minerals, amino acids, fatty acids, and sugar (glucose), which are the raw materials needed by the body to provide energy, effect repairs, and maintain functions.

Organic foods: Foods grown in soil free of chemical fertilizers, and without pesticides, fungicides and herbicides.

Outgasing: The releasing of volatile chemicals that evaporate slowly and constantly from seemingly stable materials such as plastics, synthetic fibers, or building materials.

Overload: The overpowering of the immune system due to massive concurrent exposure or to low level continuous exposure caused by many stresses, including allergens.

Parasite: An organism that depends on another organism (host) for food and shelter, contributing nothing to the survival of the host.

Pathogenic: Capable of causing disease.

Pathology: The scientific study of disease; its cause, processes, structural or functional changes, developments and consequences.

Pathway: The metabolic route used by body systems to facilitate biochemical functions.

Peak flow meter: An inexpensive, valuable tool used in measuring the speed of the air forced out of the lungs and helps to monitor breathing disorders like asthma.

Petrochemical: A chemical derived from petroleum or natural gas.

pH: A scale from 1 to 14 used to measure acidity and alkalinity of solutions. A pH value of 1-6 is acidic; a pH value of 7 is neutral; a pH of 8-14 is alkaline or basic.

Phenolics: (also known as terpenes). They are seen naturally in plants to give color and fragrance to the leaves, bark, flowers, fruits and saps. They are derivatives of benzene that are made synthetically, also to give flavor and color to foods and to help preserve them.

Postnasal drip: The leakage of nasal fluids and mucus down into the back of the throat.

Precursor: Anything that preceds another thing or event, such as a physiologically inactive substance that is converted into an active substance that is converted into an active enzyme, vitamin, or hormone.

Prostaglandin: A group of unsaturated, modified fatty acids with regulatory functions.

Radiation: The process of emission, transmission, and absorption of any type of waves or particles of energy, such as light, radio, ultraviolet or X-rays.

Receptor: Special protein structures on cells where hormones, neurotransmitters, and enzymes attach to the cell surface.

Respiratory system: The system that begins with the nostrils and extends through the nose to the back of the throat and into the larynx and lungs.

Rotation diet: A diet in which a particular food and other foods in the same "family" are eaten only once every four to seven days.

Sensitivity: An adaptive state in which a person develops a group of adverse symptoms to the environment, either internal or external. Generally refers to non-IgE reactions.

Serotonin: A constituent of blood platelets and other organs that is released during allergic reactions. It also functions as a neurotransmitter in the body.

Sick building syndrome: (Also known as building materials related illness). This term is used when one or more occupants of a building develops similar symptoms related to some indoor pollutants. Many of these symptoms involve reactions to carpets, formaldehyde, pressed woods, paints, fiber glass, tile work, chemical cleansers, leaking gas from plastic and other synthetic materials.

Steroid: A substance of naturally occurring lipid molecules such as hormones, bile acids, precursors for vitamins, and certain natural drugs; in pharmacology, a synthetic compound used to suppress the action of the immune system.

Stress: Anything that places undue strain upon normal body functions. Stress may be internal in origin (disease, malnutrition, allergic reaction), or external (environmental factors).

Sublingual: Under the tongue, method of testing or treatment in which a measured amount of an antigen or extract is administered under the tongue, behind the teeth. Absorption of the substance is rapid in this way.

Supplement: Nutrient material taken in addition to food in order to satisfy extra demands, effect repair, and prevent degeneration of body systems.

Susceptibility: An alternative term used to describe sensitivity.

Symptoms: A recognizable change in a person's physical or mental state, that is different from normal function, sensation, or appearance and may indicate a disorder or disease.

Syndrome: A group of symptoms or signs that, occurring together, produce a pattern typical of a particular disorder.

Synthesis: Combining of separate elements and substances to make a new, coherent whole.

Synthetic: Made in a laboratory; not normally produced in nature, or may be a copy of a substance made in nature.

Systemic: Affecting the entire body.

Target organ: The particular organ or system in an individual that will be affected most often by allergic reactions to varying substances.

T-cell: A white blood cell that instructs B-cells to produce antibodies in an allergic reaction, or immune reaction.

Tolerance: The capacity of the body to withstand repeated exposure without symptoms.

Tolerance threshold: The maximum amount of allergens, stress, and exposures that an individual can tolerate without having symptoms.

Toxicity: A poisonous, irritating, or injurious effect resulting when a person ingests or produces a substance in excess of his or her tolerance threshold.

Toxin: Poisonous, irritating, or injurious substance.

Vaccine: Prepared microorganism for inocculation against infectious diseases

Yin-Yang: Refers to two opposite poles of energies. Pairs of opposites—like day and night, man and woman, cold and hot.. The pairs of opposites are easier to understand when we discuss about balance and equilibrium. They are like two sides of a balance; neither side should be heavier.

Yeast: Graish-yellowing substance usually made from fermenting malt, sugar, liquor, grains, etc.

Yeast Infection: Yeast, candida, mold, fungus, all of these are opportunistic organisms, can cause life-threatening infections in immunocompromised patients. Yeast tend to cause fungaemia and focal involvement of skin and other sites. They only rarely affect persons with good host-defense.

RESOURCES

www.naet.com
NAET website for all information regarding NAET

Nambudripad Allergy
Research Foundation (NARF)
6714 Beach Blvd.
Buena Park, CA 90621
(714) 523-0800
A Nonprofit foundation dedicated to NAET research

NAET Seminars
6714 Beach Blvd.
Buena Park, CA 90621
(714) 523-8900
NAET Seminar information

Delta Publishing Company
6714 Beach Blvd.
Buena Park, CA 90621
(714) 523-0800
E-mail: naet@earthlink.net
Books on NAET

Naeter Technology
6714 Beach Blvd.
Buena Park, CA 90621
Fax: (714) 523-3068
Product available: Computer for Allergy Testing

Environmentally Safe Products
Quantum Wellness Center
Drs. Dave & Steven Popkin
1261 South Pine Island Rd.
Plantation, FL 33324
(954) 370-1900/ Fax: (954) 476-6281
E-mail: buddha327@aol.com

Cotton Gloves and other Environmentally
Safe Health Products
Janice Corporation
198 US Highway 46
Budd Lake, NJ 07828-3001
(800) 526-4237

Herbal Supplements
Kenshin Trading Corporation
1815 West 213th Street, Ste. 180
Torrance, CA 90501
(310) 212-3199

Phenolics
Frances Taylor/Dr. Jacqueline Krohn
Los Alamos Medical Center, Ste.136
3917 West Road
Los Alamos, NM 87544
(505) 662-9620

Enzyme Formulations, Inc
6421 Enterprise Lane
Madison, WI 53719
(800) 614-4400

Allergies Lifestyle & Health
205 Center Street, Ste. B.
Eatonville, WA 98328
(360) 832-0858
Health Products

Bio Meridian
12411 S. 265 W. Ste. F
Draper, UT 84020
(801) 501-7517
Computerized Allergy Testing Services

Star Tech Health Services, LLC
1219 South 1840 West
Orem, Utah 84058
(888) 229-1114
Computerized Allergy Testing Services

Apex Energetics
1701 E. Edinger, Ste. A-4
Santa Ana, CA 92705
(714) 973-7733
Homeopathic Products

Thorne Research Inc.
P.O. Box 25
Denver, ID 83825
(208) 263-1337
Herbs and Vitamins

Oxy-Health Corporation
12007 Los Nietos Road, #9
Santa Fe Springs, CA 90670
(562) 906 8888
Health Products

Clustered Solutions, Inc.
9582 Benavente St.
San Diego, CA 92129
(858) 484 6023
Clustered water

Earth Calm
3805 Windermere Lane
Oroville, CA 95965

(530) 534 9982
Dreamous Corporation
12016 Wilshire Blvd. # 8
Los Angeles, CA 90025
(310) 442 8544
Tom Wu

K & T Books
LAMC, Ste. 136,
3917 West Road
Los Alamos, NM 87544
(505) 662 9620

Wellness Program
Implementing Labs
418 Smyth Road
Ottawa, ON KIH 5A4
613-731-2772

Neuropathways EEG Imaging
427 North Canon Dr. # 209
Beverly Hills, CA 90210
(310) 276 9181

CHI/KHT
P.O. Box 5309
Hemet, CA 92544
(909) 766 1426
Health Products

Biochemical Laboratories
P.O.Box 157
Edgewood, NM 87015
(800) 545 6562

Green Healing Center C
1700 Sansom St., Ste.800
Philadelphia, PA 19103
215-751-9833
Herbs

Allergy Research Group
30806 Santana St
Hayward, CA 94544
800) 545 9960
Vitamins & Homeopathic products

QLT Corpn
3960 E. Palm Lane #9
Mesa, AZ 85215
(602) 617-1741

Life Source International
1007 Montana Ave. Ste. 125
Santa Monica, CA 90403
(310) 284 3565

Carol Sue Engleman
3944 S. W. Burma Road,
Lake Oswego, OR 97035
(503) 624-7362
Health Products

BIBLIOGRAPHY

Abehsera, Michel, Ed., *Healing Ourselves,* 1973

Ali, Majid M.D., *The Canary and Chronic Fatigue,* Life Span Press, 1995

American Medical Association Committee on Rating of Mental and Physical Impairments, *Guides to the Evaluation of Permanent Impairment,* N.P., 1971

American Psychiatric Association, *Diagnostic and Statistical Manual of Mental Disorders,* 4th ed., 2000

Austin, Mary, *Acupuncture Therapy,* 1972

Beeson, Paul B., M.D. and McDermott, Walsh, M.D., Eds., *Textbook of Medicine,* 12th edition, 1967

Bender, David, and Bruno Leone, *The Environment, Opposing Viewpoints,* Greenhaven Press, 1996

Blum, Jeanne Elizabeth, *Woman Heal Thyself,* Charles E. Tuttle Co., 1995

Brownstein, David, M.D., *The Miracle of Natural Hormones,* Medical Alternatives Press, 1998.

Brownstein, David, M.D., *The Miracle of Natural Hormones* 2nd edition. Medical 1996 Alternative Press, 1999

Brownstein, David, M.D., *Hormones and Chronic Disease,* Mdical Alternative Press, 1999

Brownstein, David, M.D., *Overcoming Arthritis,* Medical Alternative Press, 2001

Cecil Textbook of Medicine, 21st ed., 2000

Cerrat, Paul L., *Does Diet Affect the Immune System?*, RN, June 1990

Chaitow, Leon, *The Acupuncture Treatment of Pain,* Thomsons Publishers, 1984

Collins, Douglas, R., M.D., *Illustrated Diagnosis of Systematic Diseases,* 1972

Cousins, Norman, *Head First, The Biology of Hope and the Healing Power of the Human Spirit,* Penguin Books, 1990

Daniels, Lucille, M.A, and Catherine Wothingham, Ph.D., *Muscle Testing Techniques of Manual Examination,* 3rd ed., 1972

Davis, Rowland H., and Weller, Stephen G., *The Gist of Genetics,* Jones and Bartlett Publishers, 1996

East Asian Medical Studies Society, *Fundamentals of Chinese Medicine,* Paraadigm Publications, 1985

Elliot, Frank, A., F.R.C.P., *Clinical Laboratory,* 1959

Fazir, Claude A., M.D., *Parents Guide to Allergy in Children,* Doubleday & Co., 1973

Fratkin, Jake, *Chinese Herbal Patent Formulas,* Institute of Traditional Medicine, 1986

Fujihara, Ken and Hays, Nancy, *Common Health Complaints,* Oriental Healing Arts Institute, 1982

Fulton, Shaton, *The Allergy Self Help Book,* Rodale Books, 1983

Gabriel, Ingrid, *Herb Identifier and Handbook,* Sterling Publishing Co., 1980

Gach, Michael Reed, *Acuppressure's Potent Points,* Bantam Books, 1990

Goldberg, Burton and Eds. of Alternative Medicine Digest, *Chronic Fatigue and Fibromyalgia & Environmental Illness*, Future Medicine Publishing, 1998

Goldberg, Burton and Eds. of Alternative Medicine Digest, *Definitive Guide to Headaches,* Future Medicine Publishing, 1997

Goodheart, George, J., *Applied Kinesiology,* N.P., 1964

---. *Applied Kinesiology*, 1970 Research Manual, 8th ed. N.P., 1971

---. *Applied Kinesiology*, 1973 Research Manual, 9th ed. N.P., 1973

---. *Applied Kinesiology*, 1974 Research Manual, N.P., 1974

---.*Applied Kinesiology*, Workshop Manual, N.P., 1972

Gray, Henry, F.R.S., *Anatomy of the Human Body,* 27th, 34th, and 38th eds., 1961

Graziano, Joseph, *Footsteps to Better Health*, N.P., 1973

Guyton, Arthur C., *Textbook of Medical Physiology,* 2nd ed., 1961

Haldeman, Scott, *Modern Developments in the Principles and Practice of Chiropractic,* Appleton-Century-Crofts, 1980

Hansel, Tim, *When I Relax I Feel Guilty,* Chariot Victor Publishing, 1979

Harris H., M.D., and Debra Fulghum Bruce, *The Fibromyalglia Handbook*, Holt and Co., 1996

Hepler, Opal, E., Ph.D., M.D., *Manual of Clinical Laboratory Methods,* 4th ed., 1962

Heuns, Him-Che., *Handbook of Chinese Herbs and Formulae,* Vol V., 1985

Hsu, Hong-Yen, Ph.D., *Chinese Herb Medicine and Therapy,* Oriental Healing Arts Institute, 1982

---. *Commonly Used Chinese Herb Formulas with Illustrations,* Oriental Healing Arts Institute, 1982

---. *Natural Healing With Chinese Herbs,* Oriental Healing Arts Institute, 1982

Janeway, Charles A., and Travers, Paul, and Walport, Mark, and Shlomchik, Mark, *Immunobiology*, Garland Publishing, 2001

Kandel, Schwartz, Jessell, *Principles of Neural Science,* McGraw Hill, 4th ed., 2000

Kennington & Church, *Food Values of Portions Commonly Used,* J.B. Lippincott Company, 1998

Kirschmann J.D. with Dunne, L.J., *Nutrition Almanac,* 2nd ed., McGraw Hill Book Co., 1984

Krohn, Jacqueline, M.D., and Taylor, Frances A., M.A. and Larson, Erla Mae, R.N., *Allergy Relief and Prevention*, 2nd. ed, Hartley & Marks, 1996

Krohn, Jacqueline, M.D., and Taylor, Frances A., M.A., *Natural Detoxification,* 2nd. ed, Hartley & Marks, 2000

Lawson-Wood, Denis, F.A.C.A. and Lawson-Wood, Joyce, *The Five Elements of Acupuncture and Chinese Massage,* 2nd ed., 1973

Lite, Lori, *Welcome to NAET,* Lite Publishing, 2002

Lyght, Charles E., M.D., and John M. Trapnell, M.D., Eds., *The Merck Manual,* 11th ed., Merck Research Laboratories, 1966

MacKarness, Richard, *The Hazards of Hidden Allergies,* Mc Ilwain

Marohn, Stephanie, *The Natural Medicine Guide to Autism*, 1st Ed., Hampton Roads Publishing Company, 2002

Merkel, Edward K., and John, David T., and Krotoski, Wojciech A., Eds., *Medical Parasitology*, 8th. ed., W.B.Saunders Company, 1999

Milne, Robert, M.D., and More, Blake, and Goldberg, Burton, *An Alternative Medicine Definitive Guide to Headaches,* 1997

Mindell, Earl, *Vitamin Bible,* Warner Books, 1985

Moss, Louis, M.D., *Acupuncture and You,* 1964

Moyers, Bill, *Healing and the Mind,* Doubleday, 1976

Nambudripad, Devi, *Living Pain Free,* Delta Publishing Company, 1997

Nambudripad, Devi, *Say Good-bye to Illness, Spanish, 1st. ed.,* Delta Publishing Company, 1999

Nambudripad, Devi, *Say Good-bye to Illness, French, 1st. ed.,* Delta Publishing Company, 1999

Nambudripad, Devi, *Say Good-bye to Illness, English, 1st ed., 1993, 2nd. ed., 1999, 3rd. ed.,* 2002, Delta Publishing Company

Nambudripad, Devi, *Say Good-bye to ADD and ADHD,* Delta Publishing Company, 1999

Nambudripad, Devi, *Say Good-bye to Allergy-related Autism,* Delta Publishing Company, 1999

Nambudripad, Devi, *Say Good-bye to Children's Allergies,* Delta Publishing Company, 2000

Nambudripad, Devi, *Say Good-bye to Environmental Allergies,* Delta Publishing Company, 2003

Nambudripad, Devi, *Say Good-bye to Chemical Sensitivities,* Delta Publishing Company, 2003

Nambudripad, Devi, *Survivimg Biohazard Agents,* Delta Publishing Company, 2003

Nambudripad, Devi, *The NAET Guidebook,* 6th ed., Delta Publishing Company, 2001

Northrup, Christiane M.D., *Women's Bodies, Women's Wisdom,* Bantam Books, 1998

Palos, Stephan, *The Chinese Art of Healing,* 1972

Pearson, Durk, and Shaw, Sandy, *The Life Extension Companion,* Warner Books, 1984

Pert, Candace B., Ph.D., *Molecules of Emotion,* Scribner, 1997

Pitchford, Paul, *Healing with Whole Foods,* North Atlantic Books, 1993

Radetsky, Peter, *Allergic to the Twentieth Century,* Boston, Little, Brown and Co., 1997

Randolph, Theron, G., M.D., and Ralph W. Moss, Ph.D., *An Alternative Approach to Allergies,* Lippincott and Conwell, 1980

Rapp, Doris, *Allergy and Your Family,* Sterling Publishing Co., 1980

Rapp, Doris, *Is This Your Child?* Quill, William Morrow, 1991

Shanghai College of Traditional Chinese, *Acupuncture, a Comprehensive Text, 1999*

Shealy, C. Norman, M.D., Ph. D. and Caroline Myss, Ph. D., *The Creation of Health,* Stillpoint Publishing, 1993

Shima, Mike, *The Medical I Ching,* Blue Poppy Press, 1992

Shubert, Charlotte, *Burned by FlameRetardants?* Science News, Vol. 160 , 2001

Sierra, Ralph, U., *Chiropractic Handbook of Applied Neurology,* Mexico, 1956

Somekh, Emile, M.D. *The Complete Guide To Children's Allergies,* Pinnacle Books, Inc., 1979

Smith, CW, *Electromagnetic Man*: *Health and Hazard in the Electrical Environment*, Martin's Press, 1989, 90, 97

Smith CW, *Environmental Medicine*: *Electromagnetic Aspects of Biological Cycles,* 1995:9(3):113-118

Smith CW., *Electrical Environmental Influences on the Autonomic Nervous System,* 11th. Intl. Symp. on *"Man and His Environment in Health and Disease,"* Dallas, Texas, February 25-28, 1993

Smith CW., *Electromagnetic Fields and the Endocrine System,* 10th. Intl. Symp. on *"Man and His Environment in Health and Disease,"* Dallas, Texas, February 27- March 1, 1992

Smith CW., *Basic Bioelectricity: Bioelectricity and Environmental Medicine,* 15th. Intl. Symp., on *"Man and His Environment in Health and Disease,"* Dallas, Texas, February 20-23, 1997. (Audio Tapes from: Professional Audio Recording, 2300 Foothill Blvd. #409, La Verne, CA

Sui, Choa Kok, *Pranic Healing*, Samuel Wiser, 1990

Teitlebaum, Jacob, M.D., *From Fatigued to Fantastic,* 1st ed., 1996, 2nd. ed., 2001, Avery Penguin Putnam

Weiss, Jordan, M.D., *Psychoenergetics,* 2nd. ed., Oceanview Publishing, 1995

Zong, Linda, *Chinese Internal Medicine,* lectures at SAMRA University, Los Angeles, 1985

Case Histories from the Author's private practice,1984-present

Index